A
Comparative Study of Ayurveda and Treatment by Indian Drugs

Indian Medical Science Series No.-58

A Comparative Study of Ayurveda and Treatment by Indian Drugs

P.K. Chitale

Sri Satguru Publications
A Division of
Indian Books Centre
Delhi, India

Published by :
Sri Satguru Publications
A Division of :
Indian Books Centre
Indological and Oriental Publishers
40/5, Shakti Nagar,
Delhi-110007
(INDIA)

All rights reserved. No part of this work covered by the Copy-rights hereon may be reproduced or copied in any form or by any means—Graphics, Electronics or Mechanical including photocopying, microfiche reading without written permission from the publishers.

ISBN 81-7030-555-1

Second Edition : Delhi, 1997

Published by Sunil Gupta for Sri Satguru Publications a division of Indian Books Centre, 40/5, Shakti Nagar, Delhi-110 007, India and printed at D.K.Fine Art Press, Delhi-110 052

Preface

People in the villages situated far away from the hospitals and dispensaries resort extensively to the Ayurvedic system of medicine. A great many of the maladies of every day life for which doctors are consulted such us cough, colds, indigestion, ulcers, sore eyes etc. are of a minor nature and bazar medicines intelligently used have a sufficiently practical range to meet most of these maladies. These bazar medcines are easily obtainable in the bazars of almost every village and cases can be treated intelligently till regular medical aid from dispensaries become available.

Even in epidemics such as Influenza, Plague, Cholera, Relapsing Fever the prescriptions given in this book can give much relief.

The theory on which Ayurvedic system of medicine has been based and the treatment of diseases has been explained in the body of the book, and prescriptions for diseases given to avoid over-dosing by people practising this system of medicine.

Therapeutic properties of Ayurvedic drugs in use are also described in the body of the book under separate Chapter.

The Author hopes that this book may prove useful in the treatment of diseases to medical men, Vaids and Hakims working in the districts.

P.K. CHITALE,

Contents

	Pages
Chapter I Functions of Tridhatu in Ayurveda	...1
Chapter II Theory and Practice of Ayurveda	...10
Chapter III Pitt and Its Functions	...22
Chapter IV Kuff from Charaka and Sushruta	...32
Chapter V Circulation of Blood	...37
Chapter VI Composition of Body	...45
Chapter VII Diseases From वाग्भट अध्याय 2 नदान and चिकित्सा स्थान अ. 3	...50
Chapter VIII Diseases from Digestive Troubles	...62
Chapter IX From वाग्भट Vaghbhata	...86
Chapter X Worms and Germs कृमी (Krimi)	...92
Chapter XI Ayurvedic Drugs and Their Properties	...106

Chapter XII	
Diet in Ayurveda from सुश्रुत Shruta	...217
Chapter XIII	
Ear Diseases Ear-ache कर्णशूल Karnashul	...230
Chapter XIV	
Eye Diseases	...234
Chapter XV	
Diseases of Private Parts गुह्मरोग Guhya Roga	...238
Chapter XVI	
Poisons	...243
Chapter XVII	
From सुश्रुत and वाग्भट Ayurveda Surgery in Ayurveda	...248

Chapter I

Functions of Tridhatu (त्रिधातु) in Ayurveda

Ayurveda consider them as elementary unit. They are called Vat (वात), Pit (पित्त), and Kuff (कफ़). In health their functions are in equilibrium, and disordered condition causes disease. They regulate both the mental and bodily functions of the body. These three Tridhatus (त्रिधातु) carry on functions in invisible and visible forms.

Visible manifestations are seen in various secretions, body-heat, respiratory processes, deglutition, defecation, etc. Their invisible manifestations are seen in volutional impulses, body heat, respiratory processes degutition, defecation, etc.

Ayurveda further considers that the body is composed of corporal body, senses, mind, intelligence and soul.

Mind is considered to be something (some matter). Its relation to the body is very intimate. It is acted on continuously by impluses from the body without a break, only difference being that the mind is invisible. Ayurveda attributes also to these elementary invisible units of the body the properties of Satwa (सत्व), Raj (रज), and Tam (तम) that is property of consciousness, property of energy, and property of cohesion, but these three are dependent on each other. For example Vat possesses the property of stimulation in preponderance. Pitt (पित्त) property of heat, and Tam (तम) property of cohesion of atoms. Ayurveda further says that the body is made up of five elements, ether (आकाश), air (वायु), heat and light (तेज), water (आप) and earth (पृथ्वी). Wat is produced from æther and air, Pitt from light and heat and

Kuff from earth and water. As Vat is produced from the elements of ether and air, Ayurveda attributes to it the property of creative and dynamic energy. It is thus a stimulant and carries on the stimulating functions of the body by stimulating the nervous system to action.

Pitt being derived from heat and light (तेज) it contains in preponderance the quality of Satwa (सत्व) and properties of causing heat Kuff (कफ) is derived from earth and water and it contains the property of Tam (तम) that is cohesion in excess. Ayurveda attributes to this the functions of keeping the body mechanism in equilibrium and this indirectly acts on the functions of Vat (वात) and Pit (पित्त) also. It is not as yet known why oxygen gets into chemical combination with different tissue cells in the body at 98 °F and why the same combination is retarded outside the body. Ayurveda attributes this kind of function to the elementary force Kuff (कफ) in the body mechanism. Dhatus (धातु) are produced from juices after digestion. (from सुश्रुतः –

रसात् रक्त ततो मांस मासात् भेदः प्रजायते ।।
मेदसो अस्थिततो मज्झः शुक्रं तुजायते ।।

Ayurveda presumes one force (अग्नि) in each Dhatu derived from these Tridhatus (त्रिधातु). सारः तुसप्तभिः मूयो. यथास्वं पच्यते अग्निभिः ।।

अ. ह. शारीर अध्याय 3.

Agni (अग्नि) is the oxidation power in each tissues.

ओजस्तु तेजो धातुना शुक्रान्तांतां परं स्मृतम् ।।
हृदयस्थ मबि व्यापि देह स्थिति निबंधनम् ।।
यन्नाशे नियत नाशो यस्मिनं तिष्टंति तिष्टति ।।

निष्प दयन्ते यतो भावा विविधा देह संश्रया।।
ओजो विवृद्धो देहस्य तुष्टि पुष्टि बलोदय।।

अ. ह. सूत्र 11

Ayurveda attributes the process of nutrition and developement to the invisible and indirect influences of Vat (बात), Pitt (पित्त) and Kuff (कफ), and all actions and reactions during life limit and old age.

व्यस्वा षेडशात् बालं तत्र धात्विं द्वियोजसाम्।।
बृद्धिरा सप्तते मध्यं तत्र वृद्धि: पर क्षयः।।

अ. ह. शरीर 3.

Body developes up to 16, it is in middle age up to 70 and then the old age. Production, destruction and nutrition go on together. If production is in excess than destruction, body developes and after a time it becomes fully formed. After it is formed this production and destruction are in equilibrium, but after sometime the destruction predominates and the body perishes. Ayurveda says that all things are produced from five elements. (पृथ्वी) earth, (आप) water, (वायु) air, (तेज) heat and light and (आकाश) ether. These are called (पंच महाभुत) five primary elements Western science considers three states of matter, namely Solids, Liquids and Gaseous, Ayurveda considers five states viz. Solids, Liquids, Gaseous, Radient and Aetherial stages. These five elements according to Ayurveda exist in atoms (परिमाणु) and in their parts (अति परिमाणु). According to (सांख्य) philosophy these five primary elements of which the whole universe is composed have distinguishing properties.

Ether has the property of sound.
Air..............................touch
Heat.........................liquidity
Water...........................form
Earth........................solidity

and that these five kinds of properties exist in atoms Paramanu (परिमाणु) and their parts that is protons and electrons according to Western science (अतिपरिमाणु). Vedanta Philosophy still further supposes that in each atom although one of the five elements predominates, the other four still exist in (अतिपरिमाणु) that is in protons and electrons of atoms. For example in Eether which has the property of sound, this ether exists in proportion of 4 protons to 1 of electrons of other four elements (वायु) air, here Vayu (वायु) is 4 protons to 1 of other four elements. In Tej (तेज) 4 protons of tej to 1 electrons of other four elements.

(आप) water 4 protons of water to 1 electron of other four elements. (पृथ्वी) earth 4 protons of earth to 1 electron of other elements. Visible substances are derived from invisible substances and invisible substances are formed from these five elements. For example invisible earth element is derived from invisible (आप) water element. Invisible water element is derived from invisible Tej (तेज) element, invisible tej element from invisible air element, (वायु) and invisible (आकाश) from invisible ether. In this way all elements are derived from one element only. According to Western science the electrical force of the protons is positive and that round the electrons negative and the electrons of each atoms are of the same kind while Ayurveda and Vedanta Philosophy consider that the particles of (अति परिमाणु) consist of other four elements in proportion to 1 to 4 as mentioned above. Vedantha further says that it is not possible to describe (अतिपरिमाणु atiparamanu) as they are practically devoid of any weight. It is possible only to describe their qualities.

Hindu philosophy further considers that (आकाश) ether one of the five elements, which has the property of sound, has only one that property. (वायु) Air has two namely properties of sound and touch, tej (तेज) has the properties of sound, heat and touch, (आप) Ap has four sound, touch, heat and form, (पृथ्वी) earth has five, sound, touch, heat, form and cohesion. According to Western medical science dealing in endocrinology secretions from certain endocrine glands are concerned in certain mental thoughts.

Stimulus to Adrenal gland often produces angry sensations and more flow from the gland. Physiologists affirm that the body cells give off certain molecular complexes which are necessary to the growth processes and these complexes are taken up by the reproductive cells (Howell's Physiology).

Atoms are further divisible in protons and electrons. Ayurveda is in agreement with this, but further says that these protons and electrons are made up of five primary elements and Vedant philosophy still further says that in each atom although one of five elements predominates, the other four still exist. For exampl : Ether (आकाश) one of the five elements has four protons of ether to 1 of other four. (वायु) air—has four protons of wayu—to 1 of other four and so on.

According to Western science the electrical force of the protons and electrons is equal, the only difference being that the electrical force round the protons is positive and that round electrons negative. The electrons of each atoms are of the same kind while according to Vedanta these consist of other four elements in proportion of 4 protons to 1 electron.

Western medical science describes the functions of the systems of the body in physiology and that of the mind in psychology. Ayurveda describes the functions of the body and mind as one. Body is visible while mind is invisible, Ayurveda considers these as separate. Having thus described the nature of wat, pitt and kuff and their derivation from five primary elements, Ayurveda says that these forces exist in all cells and as wat is derived from the elements of ether and air, its functions are supposed to be of creative and dynamic energy. It is thus a stimulant. It stimulates the cells or atoms in the body and nervous system being most sensitive it acts on this system by exciting to action.

Pitt (पित्त) is also of the primary force in the body mechanism. It is derived from Tej (तेज) heat one of the five elements. It also exists in all the atoms and by its heating property promotes assimilation, absorption, in the systems and stimulates secretions from various glands. Kuff is derived from earth and water. It also exists in all atoms. It keeps the atoms in a condition to promote development by its cohesive power.

Having thus described the functions of (त्रिधातु) in the body and its elementary nature, Ayurveda says that the life consists of such corporal body, combined with mind and associated with Soul force.

Just as fire is produced by friction or by combination of chemical substances, so also soul associates with the elements of sperm and germ cells at the time of their union that is conception.

शुद्धे शुक्रातवे सत्वः स्वकर्म क्लेश चोदितः ।
गर्भः संप दयते युक्ती बशात् अग्नि रिवारणौः ।।
वाग्भट अध्याय 1 श्लोकं 1

Just as a ray from the sun falling upon a cow dung cake through condensed glass pyramid, remains invisible so also soul remains invisible while associating with the combined cell at the time of conception.

बिजात्मकैः महाभुतैः सूश्मैः सत्बानुगैश्चसः
मासुश्राहार रसजैः कमात् कुक्षौ विवर्धतेः

वाग्भट अध्याय 1 श्लोक 3

Elements of sperm cell from the male, elements of germ cell from the female, and the elements of the soul, together with the elements arising from the food of the mother, develop this cell gradually in the womb.

Bhagawat Gita compares this body to that of a field (क्षेत्र) kshetra and he who owns this body is called Khsetradyna (खेत्रज्ञ)

इदं शरीरं कौंतेये क्षेत्रम इति अभिधायते।
एतद्यो वेत्ती तंप्राहुः क्षेत्रश इति तत् विदः।।

भागवत गीता अध्याय 13.1

This (खेत्र) kshetra (field) consists of five elements Akash (आकाश), Vayu (वायु), (तेज) Tej, (आप) Ap, (पृथ्वी) and solid matter (Pruthwi) i.e. ether air, Radiant heat, water and solids combined with mind, intelligence, consciousness and senses. Their visible manifestations are exhibited in the feeling of will power, sensations of pain and pleasure by the body. BhagawatGita further states that this corporal body is derived from (प्रकृती) that is from nature and the qualities which it exhibits during life depend upon the preponderance of (सत्व) (Satwa) i.e. quality of Higher thinking and knowledge, (रज) i.e. quality of energy and action, and (तम) quality of ignorance.

(सत्व) Satwa produces desire for seeking happiness, Raj (रज) produces desire during life to acquire wealth and power and creates desire for action.

Tam (तम) i.e. ignorance produces desire for doing nothing i.e. keeps the body and mind during life in lower state of intellectual development, inhibits intellectual thoughts, increases desire for laziness.

ममैवांशो जीव लोके जीव भूतः सनातनः ।
मनः षष्टानी द्रियाणि प्रकृती स्थानि कर्षितः ।।
भागवत् गीता अध्याय 15 श्लोक 7.

Soul derived from me assumes form of life in the world and associates with the five elements which are combined in nature and with the mind in the body.

यतंतो योगिनश्चैनं पश्यंती आत्मन्य वस्थितं ।
यतंतो अध्य कृतात्मानों नैनं पश्यन्ती चेतसः ।।
भागवत् गीता अध्याय 15 श्लोक 11.

Only (योगी) that is those versed in concentration of thoughts becomes conscious of this soul, residing in the body, through great effort. Others do not become conscious.

द्वावि मौ पुरुषौ लोके क्षर श्रक्षर एवच ।
क्षरः सर्वाणी भुतानि कूटस्थो अक्षर उच्यते ।।
भागवत् गीता अध्याय 15 श्लोक 16.

In this world there are two things mortal and immortal, All organic things are destructible and the energy containing in them is indestructible.

उत्तमः पुरुषः त्वन्य परमात्मे त्युदाहृतः ।
यो श्लोकत्रयं आबिश्य विभर्त्यव्यय इश्वरः ।।
भागवत् गीता अध्याय 15 श्लोक 16.

Paramatma (परमात्मा) is quite separate from this. He alone is immortal pervades the whole universe and supports it.

यावत् संजायते किंचित् सत्वं स्थावर जंगमम् ।
क्षेत्र क्षेत्रज्ञ संयोगात् विद्धी भरतर्षभ ।।

Birth of any animate being is due to association of (क्षेत्र) kshetra (body and soul. भागवत् गीता अध्याय 13-33.

Just as sky though all pervading is not attached to any thing so also this soul although pervading and dominating the whole body is not in chemical combination with any thing in the body. भागवत् गीता अध्याय 13 श्लोक 32.

यथा सर्व गतं सौक्ष्म्यात् आकाशं न उपलिप्यते ।
सर्वत्रा वस्थितों देहे तथात्या नोप लिप्यते ।।

This soul is not destroyed in the mortal body.
न हन्यते हन्य माने शरीरे । भागवत् गीता अध्याय 2 श्लोक 20.

Chapter II

Theory and Practice of Ayurveda

Ayurveda considers that this body is composed of a animal (Praniz) and earthy (Parthiva) matters and both these are made of five elements Pruthvi (earthy matter), Ap (water), Tej (heat), Vayu (air) and Akash (Ether).

Pruthvi (earthy matter) contains

(1) Calcium, Sodium, Phosphorus, sulphur, magnesia and other salts etc.

(2) Ap (water) contains hydrogen and oxygen.

(3) Tej (heat) contains heat and energy.

(4) Wayu (air) contains oxygen, nitrogen and carbon etc.

(5) Akash (sky) etherial space.

Ayurveda further says that this body is made of innumerable invisible cells and is developed from oraginal seed cell which is invested with the properties of protoplasm and is fed and developed by a process of metabolism.

In Ayurveda, division has been made of various different systems by which mechanism of life is carried into दोश (Dosh), धातु (Dhatu) and मल (Mul) (दोश धातु मल मुलंहि शरीरम्) (Dosh Dhatu mul mulumhi shariram). दोश (Dosh) means generated forces in the body; धातु (Dhatu) are the generated products and मल (Mul). All things that remain to be exerted in the body after the use in the animal economy.

Ayurveda presupposes that the whole universe consists of five elements and these find entrance in the body through food and water and they increase the properties of body similar to them. All things that contain air and ether stimulate and increase those cells in the body that contain air and ether in preponderance. All things that contain dynamic or latent energy increase पित्त (Pitt) and all things that contain predominating elements of earth and water increase कफ (Kuff). The food eaten by beings is first masticated in the mouth and then it enters in the stomach. It is acted on by कफ (Kuff) and then by पित्त (Pitt). Juices of the food are separated faeces and urine and other excretory products are also separated.

(वात) (Vat) gives all power to the body mechanism. It has the power of taking the food from the mouth into stomach and from stomach into intestines. It does the digestion and separation of the juices from the excreta and through वात (Vat) all excretory processes are carried. It also carries all the juices of the food to all parts of the body.

In the body there are seven धातु (Dhatu) called रस (Ras) (juices), रक्त (Rakt) (Blood), मांस (Mans) (Flesh), मेद (Med) (Fat), अस्थी (Asthi) (Bones), मज्जा (Mujja) (Marrow) and शुक्र (Shukra) (Semen). They carry on their metabolic processes when juices of the food while circulating in the body and get into touch with these (Dhatus) each धातु (Dhatu) takes what it wants out of it digests it by its own metabolism and forms the same kinds of tissues after digestion.

In the food juices, when the properties of five elements become disproportionate disturbs the proportion of वात (Vat), (Pitt) पित्त and कफ (Kuff) and the juices are not assimilated by these seven धातु (Dhatus) and these undigested or unassimilated products cause disorder in the properties of the similar cells and containing predominant properties of the juices diminishes the properties opposite to it. Those increased properties of the cells if not counter-acted by other properties of the cells in the body find suitable nidus in any part of the body and cause what is called disease. These are internal causes of all diseases.

Diseases also arise from external causes. They don't require at the onset any increase in the properties of दोश (Dosh) in the body, and when that diseases increases दोश (Dosh) is also increased in the body which give rise to fever. In this way other five senses become in disordered condition of the body.

For example हर्ष (Harsh) (pleasure), शोक (Shoke) (Grief), (Bhaya) (Terror). These are the subjects of the mind and they act on the mind.

Wounds, fractures cause derangement of the body through external causes. Some diseases are caused through poison or unhealthy food and water and some through parents.

Charaka Samhvita says it is not possible to understand thoroughly in the body mechanism the function of वायु, पित्त and कफ (Vayu, Pitt and Kuff).

The following are the visible manifestations:

वायु (Vayu)—	Is dry, cold, light, very minute, clear movable and rough.
पित्त (Pitt)—	Slightly bitter, hot, semi-solid.
श्लेमा (Shleshma)—	Heavy, cold, sweet, and mucoid.
वायु (Vayu)—	principally resides in bladder, rectum, lumber region, shoulder and poplitieal space, and bones.

पित्त (Pitt)— in perspiration, body juices, lymph and blood and liver.

श्लेमा (Shleshma)— in lungs, head, neck, joints, stomach and fat.

वायु (Vayu)— is divided into five divisions in the body where it is preponderating.

(1) प्राण वायु (Pran Vayu)— Place of residence—Head, neck and chest.
Function— function of intelligence and mind, spitting, sneezing, respiration, deglutition.

(2) उदान वायु (Udan Vayu)—Place of residence chest, nose, neck and lower down upto navel. Function—speech, expiration, remembrance etc., etc.

(3) व्यान वायु (Wyan Vayu)—Place—Heart, and all body. Function—all the functions of the body, motor power.

(4) समान वायु (Saman Vayu)—Place—in the stomach and intestines, assimilation and digestion of food and their separation of juices.

(5) अपान वायु (Apan Vayu)—Bladder, sexual organs and rectum.
Function—defaecation, micturition and sexual production etc.

पित्त (Pitt)

(1) पाचक पित्त (Pachak Pitt)—Place—Stomach and liver: Function—digestion and separation of juices.

(2) रंजक पित्त   (Ranjak Pitt)—Liver to aid digestion.

(3) साधक पित्त   (Sadhak Pitt)—Heart—Intellectual functions.

(4) आलोचक पित्त   (Alochak Pitt)—Eyes—Vision.

(5) भ्राजक पित्त   (Bhrajak Pitt)—Skin—to keep the skin in order.

कफ (Kuff)

RESIDENCE. FUNCTION.

(1) अवलंबक कफ़ (Avalambak Kuff)—Chest—Supply of moisture in the lungs.

(2) क्लेदक कफ़ (Kleduck Kuff)—Stomach—To liquify food.

(3) बोधक कफ़ (Bodhak Kuff)—Tongue-Taste.

(4) तर्पक कफ़ (Tarpak Kuff) — Head—Satisfaction of

(5) श्लेमक कफ़ (Shlemak Kuff)—Joints—To lubricate.

वायु (Vayu) Preponderates पित्त (Pitt) in perspiration and blood and कफ़ (Kuff) in faeces and other excretions. It regulates respiration, mind, deglutition, defaecation, micturition etc.

पित्त (Pitt) regulates digestion, metabolism, sight, hunger, thirst, taste etc. and कफ़ (Kuff) stability and lubrication of the limbs (joints).

वायु (Vayu).

दोश (Dosh) धातु (Dhatu) मल (Mul).

These are the principal factors for the origin, growth and maintenance of the body, वायु (Vayu) is beneficial as it co-ordinates the functions of the body mechanism such as functions of senses, muscular co-ordination, micturition and defaecation and keeps in proportion all धातु (Dhatu) in the body and their proportionate division required in the maintenance of the body mechanism.

There are also Anabolic and Katabolic processes going on in the body both visible, and in the minute cells composing the body. In the absence of these the body cannot remain healthy. Every cell in the body is undergoing a change and this change takes place by movements and constant working. Blood circulates, muscles undergo changes and so also in the bones, there is always some change chemical and processes of destruction and building of cells.

These principle actions of the body cause absorption, assimilation and excretion. These functions are carried on by वायु (Vayu). It is an invisible force in the body and, therefore, it cannot be described properly. The principal seat in the body of वायु (Vayu) is in the large intestines and it is through it the peristaltic action in the muscular cells of large intestines continues which enable the contents of the intestines to go upwards through ascending colon and through transverse and descending colon and finally through rectum. The force that initiates this motive power in the intestines co-ordinates and keeps in proper equilibrium by causing cellular changes in the involuntary muscles of the large intestines is called वायु (Vayu). It resides here in the greater proportion as it has to do the excretion of the contents of the intestines.

कटी (Kati) (Loins) Lumbar region is second place of वायु (Vayu). It gives motive power for the excretion of urine through bladder. It acts on kidney, rectum, uterus and testis. This is called अपान वायु (Apan Vayu). If it is disordered it causes derangements in excretion of faeces, urine, uterus and foetus in pregnant women.

(3) It resides in muscles. It causes continuous Anabolic and Katabolic changes which cause movements.

(4) It also resides in the ears. It enables the processes of hearing by causing changes in the minute cells in the internal ear which are very sensitive to the vibrations of the air impinging in the ear from outside.

(5) Its fifth place is in the bones. It keeps the bones dry, hard and solid. Bones consist of marrow inside and of compact and rarified tissue and are covered by muscles and fat from outside. If this वायु (Vayu) is increased in the body or becomes disproportionate it acts on the bones. Sixth place of वायु (Vayu) is skin. It causes molecular changes in the cells and glands contained in the skin and acts and re-acts according to atmospheric changes outside the body. It coordinates the mechanism of heat regulating mechanism in the body by which the temperature of the body is kept constant and it also causes the processes of excretions of matters through the skin of matters no longer required. It also resides in the brain, scalp, lungs, heart, small intestines and rectum. It carries cellular movements between brains and skin by means of nerves whenever any disturbance is caused by vibration of air on the skin from outside or by touch of any external object or by disturbance caused by volutional or involuntary changes in the brain cells in the body. It acts on the brain, heart and on also respiration and deglutition : हृदय चेतना स्थानं मुक्तं सुश्रुत देहिणां—(Hrudayam chetana sthanum sushrut dehinam).

Ayurveda says that first vital force begins in the heat and this force then goes to the brain and causes disturbances. A sort of force is produced which is distributed throughout the body by means of nerves. It is for this reason the प्राण वायु

(Pran Vayu) is said to reside somewhere between chest and neck. It causes automatic contraction and relaxation of the heart, expansion and diminition of lungs causing processes of respiration and its effects on the brain.

उदान वायु (Udan Vayu): It resides in the lungs and its effects are in the throat, nose and diaphragm and abdomen. It produces a force which principally carries expansion and relaxation of the elastic portion of the lungs:

उरस्थान मुदानस्य नासानाभी गलांश्चेरेत ।
नाक्प्रवृत्ती प्रयन्त्तोजी बलवर्ण स्मृती क्रिय ।। :

(Ursthan mudanasya nasanabhi galanschartet,)
Nakprakruti praytonji balanwarna smruti kriya.)

It causes speech, source of power and promotes remembrance. Movements of lungs carries also the cellular movements in the body mechanism. Respiration is caused by both प्राण वायु and उदान वायु (Pran Vayu and Udan Vayu).

व्यान वायु (Vyan Vayu): It resides in heart.

व्यानो हृदिस्थित! कृत्स्न देहचारी महाजवः

(Vyano hrudistitha—Rrutsne dehchari mahajawah)

It moves throughout the body. It co-ordinates all muscle movements of the body. Heart is one of the most important organ in the body. It circulates the blood to all parts and produces चैतन्य (Chaitanya) (Life). All the actions of the body are due to रक्त (Rakt) (Blood). रस धातु ((Ras Dhatu) internal metabolism and चैतन्य (Chaitanya) sensitiveness to actions and reaction. समान वायु (Saman Vayu): It resides in the small intestines.

समानो अग्नि समीपस्थ कोष्टे चरती सर्वतः
अन्न गृणहाती पचती विवेचयती मुंचती।।

(Samanoa agni samipastha koshte charati sarvata)
(Annum grunhati pachti vivechayati munchati)

It is near the jatharagni in the small intestines and pervades the whole of the small intestine. It takes up the food, digests it and aids in the assimilation and separation of the food juices and assists in the evacuation of excreta. Food after having entered the small intestine from आमशय (Amashaya) (Stomach)—It is acted upon by the juices from the bodies in the small intestines which aids in the digestion and separation from the assimilable parts, the food particles that are of no use to the animal economy and which are required to be excreted. This is effected by disturbance produced by this वायु (Vayu).

Fifth is अपान वायु (Apan Vayu). It resides in the lumbar region and aids in defaecation, micturition etc. These are the functions of what is called वायु (Vayu) in the Ayurveda. In fact it has the property of causing irritability and consequent changes of contraction of expansion in the body cells by its own changes caused by response to stimuli either in the body such as cell or from outside influences. When this is not in proportion or in order in the body it causes many disorders.

(1) पाद शुल (Pad Shul): Burning sensation in the hands and feet.

(2) विपादिका (Vipadika): Dryness in the hands and feet.

(3) सुप्तपादता (Supta Padat): Anaesthesia of the feet.

(4) जानु भेद (Janu Bhed): Pains in the joints.

(5) उरूसाद (Urusad): Anaesthesia of the knees.

(6) पांगुलच (Panguluch): Paralysis of the legs.

(7) गुदाति (Gudati): Pains at the anus.

From the description given above it will be seen that the functions of the वायु (Vayu) as described in Ayurveda more or less resemble functions of nervous system. It is considered as one of the vital forces that principally act on the nerve protoplasm causing disturbance by its property of response to stimuli in the body cells while in contact with them. It is said to be composed of five elements of which body itself is composed. The disturbance is produced in these elements by its action and reaction on the body cells and by outside influences which evolves into some sort of force which disturbs the delicate protoplasm of the nerve tissue. This either depresses or excites the coarser structures in the body.

According to Western medical science the nervous system in the body is composed of number of centres with an excitable surface on one side and organs of force on the other. Disturbance on the excitable surface causes a molecular change in the associated nerve terminations. This is conducted by an apparent nerve through the posterior root ganglion to the spinal cord from which it may be transmitted to the brain as a sensation or may be reflected again through efferent tracts and nerves as an impulse to the organs of force such as muscles, organs, glands etc. The functions of nervous substance however are automatic and reflexive. The highest centres are in the convolutions. Automatic and reflex centres are in the cerebellum and medulla and cord and these are associated to each other by tracts which conduct associates and co-ordinate the impulses, Peripheral ganglia of the sympathetic nerve are chiefly automatic in action. All the organs in the body are governed by centres in the medulla and cord and they are constantly influenced by impressions reacting them from all sides. Viscera moreover have intrinsic local ganglia acting automatically but controlled to some degree by the higher centres.

Sensation is a consciousness of the brain referrable to an impression or impulse received from the periphery. Which if travelled upwards becomes perception.

Motion is caused by impulse arising in the contractile motor area transmitted through lower centres and cord through motor nerves to terminal portions of nerves in the muscles.

Consciousness resides in psychical areas of the cerebral convolutions while sleep is associated with diminished metabolism of grey matter.

वायु (Vayu): In Ayurvedic medicine is considered to be something which is invisible and which cannot be felt. It consists of atoms. रूप रहित स्पर्शवान् वायु– (Rup Rahit sparshwan vayu) with supplies motion to the various system in the body. It is derived from the word वा (Va). It supplies this invisible motion to carry atoms in the various systems in the body.

Charaka says: स्रोतसामेव समुदायं पुरुष मिच्छंति— (Srotasamew samudayum purushamichanti) and वायु (Vayu) consisting of atoms, it has a constant movement. These atoms reside in atmosphere and body consists of five elements and, therefore, of atoms: पंच महा भूत शारीरि समवाय स्वरूपि (Panch maha bhuta shariri sam waya swarupi). In it there are visible and invisible entrances.

Visible entrances are mouth, anus, nose that is passage for taking food, passage for excreta and passage for air.

There are also invisible pores. These are filled in with वायु (Vayu): and as its atoms possess power of motion they act and react on the atoms and cells composing the body producing motion in the body. In these actions natural activity of the body is carried out and when from external or internal causes these natural actions and reactions are in any way hindered or exaggerated it produces a disease.

वायु (Vayu) when acted upon by पित्त (Pitt) produces the heated sensations in the body, thirst, colic dizziness, burning sensation in the stomach, mouth and desire to eat cold things, when acted on by कफ़ (Kuff) it produces coldness, heaviness and desire to take exercise and to eat hot and dry food, when acted of by blood it produces itching sensation in the skin, irritation of the skin and pimples, when acted on by muscles tingling sensation in the hands and feet and local inflammation on the skin and when by bones tingling sensation all over the body, coldness, and when acted on by fat yawning and pains in the bones and when acted on by food—stomach, colic and when acted on by urine—difficulty in micturation.

All these disorders are caused by वायु (Vayu) by irritating the nerves supplying those parts.

Chapter III

Pitt and Its Function

Pitt (पित्त) is derived from the word Tap (तप) to heat. The word Pitt signifies heat. It aids in digestion, assimilation.

Definition of Pitt — पित्तंसस्नेह तक्ष्णोष्णां लघु विस्यं सरं द्रवं ।।

(Pittam sasnahum tekshnoshna laghu wisyam sarum drawam)

It is a force which regulates the secretions in the body. Its external manifestation is seen in the secretions and is described as such. It is slightly acid, liquid, hot and a little oily.

It regulates the secretions from various glands in the body such as peptic and acid glands in the stomach and intestines and from liver and pancreas secretions.

(1) Its effect is principally seen in the glands near Umbilicus. It is a factor which aids in assimilation and digestion of the food in the intestines and maintains body heat and metabolism.

नाभि रामाशयः स्वेदोलसीका रूधिरं रसः

हक् स्पर्शनंच पित्तस्य नाभिरत्र रिााशेशतः

(Nabhiramashaya swedolasika rudhirnm rasa

Druk sparshsnch pittasya Nabhiratra wisheshta)

(2) Its effect is produced on the stomach and liver and acts on the food.

(3) It is seen in blood. It helps to keep the blood in liquid form and maintains its normal heat. Its effects are

seen in fat and lymph. It is also found in (रस धातु) Ras Dhatu (body juices).

Ras Dhatu (रस धातु) is formed by mixture of food and juices and intestinal juices and bile. Its effect is seen in heart. It helps to keep that organ into proper heat by causing contraction and relaxation of the heart which helps to maintain the blood in proper fluid form. It is also found in eyes which helps to keep the vision. It is also found to some extent in the skin. It helps to regulate the heat of the body. In fact Pitt can be described as some power acting on the glands in the body which has the power to digest all substance eaten for the maintenance of the body heat. It pervades in all parts of the body and its effects are visible in the intestinal tract where the process of digestion is greatest and longest but it also exists in other different parts composing the animal mechanism and when this is not in order it produces disorders.

(1) Osh (ओष): Tingling sensation on one particular part.

(2) Plosh (प्लोष): Blister on the skin.

(3) Dah (दाह): Burning sensation all over the body.

(4) Wadwathu (वदवथु): Inflammation on one part of the body.

Again when liver is deranged digestion and assimilation are disturbed which give rise to bitter and acid taste in the mouth and foul smell.

These are due to excess of Pitt in the upper part of intestines.

Great thirst: This is due to excessive heat caused by disordered and excessive secretions of glands containing good deal of latent heat.

Atrupti (अतृप्ति): This is due to excess and immediate digestion of food in the stomach by disordered action of Pitt, when it is in excess in the eyes it produces darkness before the eyes.

Burning in the throat and stomach and acid eructations are due to disorders of Pitt and symptoms of Amla Pitt (आम्ल पित्त) are indigestion, fatigue, watering in the mouth and sensation of vomiting, acidity in the mouth.

Atisweda (अतिस्वेद): Profuse perspiration. This is due to disorders of Pitt in the blood. By the excess of heat in the body it makes the blood more fluid excess of water in the blood gets out through the system from the pores of the skin.

Ang-gandh (अंग गंध): Foul smell from the skin is due to undigested and unassimilated products passing out of the blood through the skin.

Sore eyes, burning sensation in the skin, rectum and in urine are all due to production of excess of heat in the body. These conditions are due to disordered action of Pitt in the blood circulating to these parts.

Eruptions on the body are due to heated condition of blood owing to retarded circulation in the skin and so also greenish, yellowish and reddish pigmentation of skin.

Different degenerated conditions of blood producing jaundice are also due to this.

Small intestine is one of the place where this Pitt (पित्त) acts on food through bile and some of the juices of the food are absorbed which go to make blood.

When Pitt (पित्त) is produced in excess in the body it retards the various functions of the organs giving rise to several diseases in the system.

According to Western science the process of absorption begins from the food we eat. In the mouth food is masticated it is mixed with mucus and saliva and its starchy constituents are partly converted into maltose and others are dissolved. Flow of saliva is regulated by the nerves.

Saliva lubricates the bolus and imparts to it a faintly alkaline reaction. Food then descends in the stomach through gullet. Gastric digestion is mainly effected by the gastric juice. It owes its solvent and chemical powers to pepsin which is acted upon by hydrochloric acid and resolves into lipase and rennin and this is assisted by the churning movements of the stomach concentrating towards the pylorus which alternately opens and contracts and this product of gastric digestion (chyme) is gradually transferred towards the duodenum.

Proteids become soluble, diffusible peptones, sugar converted into dextrose and laevulose fats decomposed. Putrefactive organisms in food are destroyed by acids. Chyme passes out of the stomach with an acid reaction and it is acted by an alkaline fluid, a mixture of pancreatic juice bile and enteric juice. Pancreatic juice contains three ferments trypsin which acts on proteids and splits it up into amino acids such as leucin, tyrosin and alanin. Diastase ferment converts starch into maltose and dextrin.

Lipase converts fats into glycerine and fatty acids.

Enteric juices contain trypsin a proteolytic ferment converting proteins into peptones. Enterokinase activator of trypsogen and ferments converting sugar into glucose.

Bile aids the digestion of fats precipitates proteids stimulates peristaltic movements and lessens intestinal putrefaction, muscular movements of duodenum are partly progressive and partly churning. The main absorption products of gastric and pancreatic digestion commence in the duodenum and is continued in the small intestines. In the upper part of intestine the food intimately mixed with the pancreatic biliary and intestinal juices continues to undergo digestion and it acted on by bacteria by which carbohydrates are converted into Lactic, Butyric and Carbonic acid Proteins are resolved into Phenol derivatives, Amino acids into toxic amines, fats into lower acids, Butyric, Valeric. The food absorption commences from duodenum and is mostly accomplished in the jejunum and illium. It is not absorbed finally by osmosis. Epithelium of the intestines selects what is to be absorbed for the system in which action under lying leucocytes also take part. Proteins are absorbed in the form of amido acids. Carbohyrates are absorbed as monosaccharides. Proteins, carbohydrates, salts and water enter the portal circulation. Rate of absorption depends on the rapidity of intestinal circulation and on the osmotic tension of intestinal contents as compared with blood plasma and on the condition of the absorbtive power of the intestinal mucus membrane. Fats are split up into glycerine and fatty acids and are absorbed by the Epithelium of intestines and they are resynthetized into fat and transferred to the lacteals. By the time the intestinal contents reach the colon the digestive products are mainly absorbed. Excretion is very active in the small intestines.

The watery secretions are separated from the blood partly by osmosis from the vessels and partly by the glands. Intestinal epithelium also excretes all toxins. In the large intestines absorption of the food residue continues but as the transmission of contents is slower, more water is absorbed and faeces become formed. Consistency of the faeces depends upon the activity of absorption, excretion and rate of transit. The transit of the contents of the intestines is effected by peristalsis. It is the result of co-ordinated reflex action. The function is automatic and brought into action by mechanical stimulation of food and influenced in activity by muscular exercise, emotions and sensations.

The whole system is influenced by evacuation:

1. A certain amount of water is removed from circulation.
2. Bile is swept out and liver is stimulated.
3. Certain solids excreted by Epithelium of the intestinal wall and fit to be excreted are thrown out.
4. Circulation of the blood in the abdomen is disturbed.
5. Blood circulates more freely in liver and portal system and heart is thus relieved.
6. Circulation in the brain is diminished.
7. Circulation through renal artery and kidney is increased and pressure in the ureter is lowered.

The substances that enter the liver through portal vein are the products of digestion. Constituents of proteins, glucose, salts, a trace of fat amido acids and abundant water. Amino acids are hydrolysed by hepatic cells nitrogenous portion is turned into urea and non-nitrogenous portion is returned to the blood and it serves as source of energy. Glucose is converted into glycogen by liver cells and as it is required glycogen is again transformed mainly into sugar by means of enzyme and partly into fat and gluco protein. This decomposition may be increased by nervous influences. Liver also carries on fat metabolism. Fat is stored in connective tissue and by ferment it is converted into fatty acids and glycerol which are carried to the liver and where it is further decomposed into simpler fatty acids—caproic and butyric and which are oxidized by the tissues into carbon dioxide and water. Liver also stores alkaloids and metallic salts from the intestines.

Bile secretion is formed in response to the chemical stimulus of secretine. Bile pigment results from decomposition of Haemoglobin. Bile in the intestines precipitates peptonized protein, disolves fatty acids and resins and augments peristalsis. Biliary salts are reabsorbed from the bowels and carried back to the liver and there converted into cholates and once more secreted and discharged into the bowels.

While this is going on intramolecular chemical changes occur in living tissues while in action in presence of blood. The blood that passes through muscles becomes venous that it loses oxygen a small quantity of ammino acids and other elements of plasma and takes up waste products. When a muscle contracts certain chemical substances are produced namely carbonic acid, water, sarcolactic acid, amonia, uric acid, urea and other nitrogenous bodies. This process of double decomposition is going on in every cell and organ of the body both constructive and destructive. Normally these processes are more or less in equilibrium. The products coming from food are balanced by the excretion of carbon, nitrogen and water in the urine, faeces and breath. Nitrogen excretion is wholly excreted, carbon is retained in the form of fat to some extent which is excreted again during muscular work. In the liver glycogen is decomposed into glucose and in the tissues into lactic acid and by further oxidation into carbon dioxide and water glycoromic acid is decomposed into water and carbon dioxide in the muscle tissue by an enzyme secreted from the pancreas. Fat absorbed through intestines passes into the lacteales and blood to the cells of adipose tissue and is split up into fatty acid and glycerine by ferment and there again resynthetized and stored for use as required. Fat is used up during muscular exercise. It is carried to the liver and decomposed into lower acids. Butyric, hydroxybutyric and caproic and by successive oxidation into tissues, into ascetic acid and then into carbon dioxide and water. Carbohydrates can also be formed into fats by the liver. Fats and carbohydrates produce muscular energy and heat, proteins are necessary for tissue waste. A small portion of amino acids is used by tissue cells to reconstruct tissue proteins and they are then catabolized into ammonia, cretinin and urea. This is called endogenous metabolism. The remainder are deamidized by liver and are excreted as urea by the kidneys. Similarly, purin substances derived from nuclei are decomposed into tissues, into uric acid either by exogenous or endogenous process. Even uric acid if excessive may be broken up in the liver into allentoin and urea but normally it is excreted as urates. Metabolism like digestion is associated with intracellular ferment. Intimate protoplasmic changes are the basis of vital force and are controlled by nervous system, by trophic centres lying in the brain and spinal cord and spinal ganglia with afferent and efferent trophic fibres and also in part by vasomotor system. Endocrine glands are the following:

Pituitary, suprarenal, thyroid, parathyroid and thymus. They have important influence in the maintaining of growth and metabolism of the body system and in regulating the normal function of the organs in the body.

Body Heat: It is produced in every act of vital energy and is lost in the surrounding medium. In the warm-blooded animals certain amounts of heat is accumulated in the system. This amount of heat is constant. Any excess is lost in the surrounding air and exactly balances the production. Body heat in human beings is 98.4 °F. Temperature of the body is controlled by nerve mechanism. It consists of governing centre, heat regulating centre in the brain. Afferent nerves from skin, mucus membrane carry impressions of heat and cold to them. These impressions are carried to the cortex of the brain causing sensation of temperature, and to sweat centres in the cord and metabolic or trophic centres in the spinal cord and brain. These centres are in relation with cardiac, respiratory and vasomotor centres, and they affect the circulation, blood pressure etc. so as to regulate the body heat to such an extent as to keep the constant temperature by increased or diminished production of heat. Heat from the body is lost through skin and lungs by perspiration and increased respiration. Sweat glands in the skin are excretory glands of water, salts, and for nitrogenous products. They are influenced by nerve mechanism : centres of which are situated in the spinal cord. Now Pitt as said above is derived from the word, Tap (तप्) to heat. It is also called Pachak Ras (पाचक रस) digestive juice. In the liquid from it is considered to be the secretions of the organs and endocrine glands that is to say the heat producing properties preponderate in those fluids which are capable of producing chemical action on the food in the digestive tract and alteration in body cells producing absorption and production of heat. This process is constantly going on in the abdomen. Ayurveda, therefore, supposes that the chief centres of this production of body heat is near Nabhy (नाभी) i.e. somewhere near the Umbilicus and Amashaya (आमाशय) and Yakrit (यकृत) stomach and liver and Ras-Dhatu (रस धातु) a mixture of food and intestinal juices. Pitt (पित्त) is also required in the blood to keep its proper heat. Ayurveda, therefore, supposes that Pitt is second fundamental principle in which processes of life are carried on by maintaining heat by constant changes in the body cells. Those juices that assist in assimilation and digestion such as bile etc. are considered to be Pitt because those juices contain properties of causing chemical action and cellular changes which go to produce heat in the system. In fact the word Pitt includes all the processes of assimilation, digestion, metabolism and heat regulating apparatus. These processes are further acted on by Vat (वात) which carries on the functions of central nervous system and which is said to supply invisible motion through atoms in the various systems in the body.

Chapter IV

Kuff from Charaka and Sushruta

Ayurveda describes this as follows:

Snigdh shito gurumandum lakhne mrutsne sthir kuff.

स्निगधः शीतो गुरुमंदः लक्ष्णे मृत्स्नः स्थिरः कफ ॥

अ. हृ. रू. स्था.

It is that force in the body, which regulates the properties of cohesion, adhesion and lubrication. It is through it the whole body is kept together and has a form. Ayurveda describes this as Shlema (श्लेमा). It exists in all parts of the body and is manifested in cells and atoms composing it. Only the physical properties of this power as seen and felt are described above. Visible manifestation of this, is cold, oily, heavy, mucoid and stable. It is mostly seen in its fluid form in the following parts of the body:

Chest, throat, head, joints, stomach, blood, fat, and nose.

उरः कंठशिरः क्लोम पवार्णयामाश योरसः
मेदो प्राणांच जिव्हाच ऋफस्य सुतरा मुरः

अ. हृ. रू. स्था

श्लेमास्थिरत्व स्निग्घत्व संघिबध क्षमादिभिः

अ. हृ. रू. स्था.

Functions

It has the property of bringing steadiness to the body and keeps the joints in position. Its principal function is in the chest and especially in the lungs. It facilitates the expansion and contraction of lungs during respiratory processes by steadying and keeping it in proper form. When process of respiration is going on normally it is produced in moderate quantity by the glands in the bronchi and blood in the lungs. When digestion is disorderd this power of producing kuff is also increased by vitiated juices in the blood from intestinal canal.

This is also produced in the throat to keep it moist and to facilitate deglutition of food. It also exists in the head to keep the brain cool and fit to carry out the normal brain functions of the body. It keeps all the joints in position. It is produced by the glands in the stomach to make the food more liquid and fit for digestion. It also exists in fat to keep its lubricant property. It exists in the tongue and facilitates the formation of bolus of food and its deglutition. Besides these places it exists in all cells of the body in very minute quantity to keep them in cohesion and prevents the process of excessive wear and tear and oxidation. When cough is produced in excess the following symptoms arise:

Loss of appetite, lassitude, sleepiness, sense of fatigue, sense of heaviness in the limbs, laziness, sweetness in the mouth, sticky sensation in the mouth, eructations, coughing, diarrhoea, dimunition of heart's action, loss of heat, puffiness in the skin, paleness over the skin, pale and whitish appearance over the skin, eyes, urine and faeces.

Organs in the body are dependent on each other and when one is in disorder others are also affected by it. When cough is in excess in the lungs it produces at first bronchitis and later on Asthma. Excess of cough in the lungs disorders the proper expansion and contraction of the lungs and the aeration of blood. If one eats articles in diet which have property of production of cough in excess it produces different diseases in proportionate to its accumulation in different parts. For example if produced in excess in the intestines it produces disordered actions of the bowels and production of all other diseases arising from it. By increase of cough breathlessness is originated, so also when it is produced in excess in the head it produces sensation of lassitude, laziness, heaviness in the limbs etc. According to the Western science the act of respiration consists of inspiration and expiration which is governed by the respiratory centre. This centre is influenced by increasing of body temperature and by impulses from the brain and reflex impressions conveyed by all sensory nerves and particularly by those from nose and mouth. The respiratory centre is usually active and the act of inspiration is normally checked by an inhibitory impulse by passing up the respiratory vagus fibres at the moment the respiration reaches its height. Normal respiration is a passive act in recoil. In forced breathing a forced inspiration sets up expiratory impulses which excite the respiratory centre, vagus nerve controls the rate of inspiration. Sensory impressions received from the lungs are not normally perceptible by an individual but in diseases they give rise to feeling of distress, oppression or actual pain. Apart from nervous control the respiratory centre is extremely sensitive to any increase in carbonic acid tension which causes increased depth of respiration. It responds also to decreased oxygen tension but only when it falls much beyond the normal. The deficiency in oxygen may arise by (1) insufficient oxygen pressure in the blood (2) lack of haemoglobin (3) by impairment in circulation such as in chronic heart disease in haemorrhages, shock and syncopy.

As respiratory centre responds immediately to lack of oxygen by increased breathing when this is associated with excess of carbon dioxide the condition is automatically relieved, but if there be no excess of carbon dioxide the increased breathing eliminates more carbon dioxide so that its concentration in the blood is reduced, that is less oxygen is dissociated from oxyhaemoglobin in the tissues. (2) Respiratory centre is deprived of its normal stimulus. This oxygen want is called Anoxaemia. The temperature of the air, moisture, the pressure of the air also affect the respiratory centre. Red corspucles and plasma of the blood modify the respiratory activity and so also the circulation and also by the ciliary action of the cells in the respiratory passages. The mucus secretion of the glands in the bronchi also affect the respiratory activity. The flow of saliva is regulated by nervous impulses. It acts on the food and enzyme diastase splits starch and glycogen into maltose and dextrin which is subsequently converted into dextrose. Saliva also lubricates the bolus of food and imparts to it faintly alkaline reaction which continues conversion of starch into sugar until the acid permeates the bolus in the stomach. Some excretions are also thrown out by the glands in the mouth.

Muscular acts of mastication are guided by affarent impressions and by the will. Disorders of secretion of the mouth include disturbances in the quantity of saliva and mucus. Saliva becomes deficient in indigestion and in fevers and in diabetesec ausing dryness in the tongue. Similar condition is induced in depressing condition such as fear or grief. Reflex action of increased saliva occurs in vomiting and in some cases of gastro-intestinal disorder. Derangement of excretions of the mouth causes bad taste and unpleasant odour of the breath due to digestive derangements and bacterial infection of the mouth, teeth and gums. Another cause of indigestion is due to imperfect mastication and insufficient salivation. Cough (Kuff) as said above increases the secretions of the glands in the mouth and in the lungs and thus helps in the respiration and digestion. Ayurveda then considers the existence of these principal factors that exist in the body. त्रिधातु (Tri-Dhatu) (Vayu, Pitt and Kuff), Sapta Dhatu सप्तधातु and Mul मल may be called anabolic products cell metabolism and catabolic products. Tridhatus are Vatt, Pitt and Kuff.

Dhatus are seven—they are Rasa रस, Rakt रक्त (Blood), मांस (Mussle), Med मेद (Fat), Asthi अस्थी (Bones), Mujja मज्जा (Marrow) and Shukra शुक्र (Semen).

They carry on metabolic processes in the cells generating energy, action and body heat etc. Mul मल are the excretory processes of the body, through pores of the skin, lungs, kidneys urine and faeces. These i.e. Vayu, Pitt and Kuff in the process of life get deranged by external and internal causes and vitiate Dhatu and Mul and thus produce various ailments.

Chapter V

Circulation of Blood

Blood is formed out of the juices absorbed the food in the intestines after being acted upon by juices of live and spleen.

यांभिरिदं शरीर मा राम इव जल हारिणीभिः ।
केदार इव कुलयाभिरुप स्निह्यते अनुगृह्यतेचः ॥
(सु. शा.)

All the body parts are irrigated by the vessels that carry the blood. Ayurveda knew the dynamic law of circulation.

व्यानेन रस धातुर्हि विक्षेपोचित कर्मरण
युगपत्क्षिप्यते अजस्त्रं देहे विक्षिप्यते सदा
अष्टांग हृदय
शारीर अध्याय 3

Wyan Vayu (व्यान वायु): Wyan Vayu contracts the heart and throws the blood in the arteries and all over the body and then the heart dilates and blood enters the heart through the veins.

तेन मूलेन महता महा मूला मतादश ।
ओजो वहा शरीरे अस्मिन् विश्रम्यन्तो समन्ततः ॥
येना जसा वर्तयन्ति प्रीणीताः सर्व जन्तवः ।
यदृते सर्व भूतानां जीवितं नाव तिष्ठते ॥
चरक सूत्र अ. 30.7

Maha-Mula means heart. From the heart arteries carry blood to all parts of the body and all parts of the body are fed by the blood through the arteries and in its absence it is not possible for the animal to live. Further on it says:

यत्सार मादौ गर्भस्य यत्तद्गर्भ रसाद्रसः
संवर्तमानं हृदयं समाविशार्तयत्पुराः
चरक अध्याय 30-9

Blood supports foetus and after supporting it again comes back to the heart of the mother.

Respiration.—

नाभिस्थः प्राण पवनः स्पृष्ट्वा हृत्कमलांतरम् ।
कंठाष्दहि विनिर्याति पातुं विष्णु पदामृतम् ॥
पीत्वा चांबर पीयूषं पुनरायाती वेगत ।:
प्रीणयन् देह मखिलं जीवचं जठरानलम् (शारंगधर)
प्रथम खंड अध्याय 5

Vayu (वायु): From above navel region and air in the lungs go out of the throat and taking up oxygen (विष्णु पदामृत) Vishnoo Padamrut and throwing out the vitiated matter it enters again the system and thus keeps the body in a pleasant condition. Blood supplies all necessary bodies to the tissues and takes out all that is necessary. This is called Danopadan-Kriya (दानोपदान क्रिया) (Metabolism). This forms, Sapta Dhatu and on it depends the health. This metabolism again depends on food, air, water, exercise and digestion when caused in a proper form in the body.

According to the Western science blood consists of plasma, red and white corpuscles. It carries proteins, fats, sugar, salts and different internal secretions and the products of vital processes namely carbonic acid, water, urea, uric acid, salts and other substances. It also provides immunity against pathogenic micro-organisms. It contains sodium bicarbonate and phosphate which forms loose combinations with carbonic acid formed out of metabolism in the tissues and thus resist increase of carbonic acid gas in the blood. It supplies oxygen to the tissues which remains in free solution about 2 p.c. and as this amount diminishes it is replenished by the giving off of oxygen from the heamoglobin in which increased carbon doxiode tension of the tissue assists. Functions of white corpuscles are partly nutritive i.e. glycolytic and partly assistance in procuring immunity by being phagocytic. Co-agulation of plasma is brought about by the conversion of fibrinogen into soluble fibrine by enzyme thrombine derived from the disintegration of leucoeytes tes and blood plates by action on it of two agents a harmone derived from the tissue and calcium salts. Red corpuscles are the carriers of oxygen to the tissues. The combination of oxygen and heamoglobin being loose. In the lungs where the oxygen tension is high heamoglobin takes up the gas. In the tissues where the tension of carbon dioxide is high it gives up oxygen. The red corpuscles contain phosphorus and various salts. Red blood corpuscles are derived from the erythro blasts of bone marrow and are ultimately broken up to form pigments of the bile, faeces and urine. Heart drives a certain amount of blood from the circulatory system in a given time. The heart contracts by virtue of the properties of cardiac muscle for rhythmic contraction. Stimulus is provided by the salts of blood. Sodium salts of the blood maintain the osmotic condition promoting excitability and contractility. Calcium salts maintain tone and contractility and potassium induces relaxation in diastole contraction which starts at the sino-auricular node passes through the auricle to the ventricle travels first to the papillary muscles and then to the ventricle. Auriculoventricular node is also capable of starting a rhythm of its own. This contraction of the heart also gives rise to electric currents. Positive wave starts from the auricle and is succeeded by contraction of auricle and it is followed by electrically quiescent period followed by second positive wave starting the contraction of ventricle and is followed by second period of quiescent. The movements of the heart are regulated by vagous nerve and by sympathetic from the first four dorsal nerves. Stimulus of vagus centre nerve ganglia or endings leads to prolongation of diastole and stimulation of sympathetic results in the acceleration of tone contractility and conductivity of muscular fibres. Cardiac centre is in the medulla and affected by sensory impulses from nose, throat, lungs, skin, and viscera and also affected by psychical factors such as fright. The vagus centre is also affected by blood supply. High blood pressure stimulates it and so also low blood pressure and venous blood slows the heart. The heart is also supplied by sensory nerves by the vagus stimulation of which starts pain in the precardia or to the left side. The arteries are system of branching tubes composed mainly of involuntary muscular fibres and controlled by vasomotor centres in the medulla and by subsidiary centres in the cord by vasoconstrictor and vaso-dilator nerves. The tone of the arteries is normally maintained by stimulating action on the vasoconstrictor ending by internal secretions from adrenalin, pituitrin and thyroid. Certain organs such as brain and lungs have no vasomotor nerves controlling their vessels as they require an amount of blood at constant pressure. Vasomotor centre is stimulated by low blood pressure, venous condition of blood and reflexly by stimulation of sensery nerves and by psychical factors such as fear etc., and its activity is diminished by fear and impressions from the viscera. It is also affected by the affarent impression from the heart and aorta. These are conveyed by sensory fibres of vagus which join the superior laryngeal. Impressions of over distension or distress of heart are conveyed by the depressure nerve of the heart to the vasomotor centre resulting in the relaxation of the arteries which lessens the peripheral resistance to relieve the heart. General blood pressure depends (1) on the force of the heart-beat (2) on the elastic recoil of aorta (3) on the total quantity of blood. Capillaries distribute the blood to the tissues. Leucosites and plasma of blood flow out through the thin walls, gas exchanges take place and besides capillaries promote the return of the products of metabolism from the tissues into the blood stream. They are not contractile but the blood flow is affected by alterations in their lumen and changes in the venous pressure.

Veins—Convey the blood to the heart. They are provided with valves. They are influenced by posture, muscular movement, respiratory activity and the volume of blood passing through them. In inspiration negative pressure in the chest dilates the great vesels and sucks more blood into them. Increased force of the heart beat reduces venous pressure by emptying auricles and increasing pulmonary circulation. High peripheral resistance lowers the pressure. On the other hand if the heart is unable to overcome great resistance and is incompletely emptied back pressure leads to increased venous pressure and so also increased volume of blood. High venous pressure promotes transudation from the capillaries.

Pulse—Heart drives a certain amount of blood through the whole length of circulatory system in a given time, this system is already full. This contraction increases the tension in the arteries by stretching the arteries. Intermitent action of the heart, peripheral resistance and arterial elasticity effect a constant flow of blood through the capillaries and veins. Blood pressure is highest in the arteries. The wave raised by each contraction of the heart is known as pulse. It consists of sudden rise, slight fall and another small rise and fall. It varies from 70 to 80 beats per minute. It is best felt at the radial artery at the wrist. The up stroke represents the contraction of ventricles driving blood into the aorta and thereby causing a wave which is rapidly transmitted to the peripheral arteries. The apex of this strike is known as percussion wave. Of the elevation in the course of down stroke the most constant is dicrotic wave due to reflected wave from the closed aortic valves and from the walls of aorta. It is preceded by a slight depression aortic notch which marks the end of contraction of heart. This is followed by 2 or 3 slight undulations there are only elastic elevations. Various pulse—this occurs in various conditions of diseases although in some cases it appears to be a normal phenomenon. *Circulation in the kidneys*—large renal artery direct branch from abdominal aorta where blood pressure is high supplies the kidney on each side. The blood pressure in the kidney substance (Glomerulus) is high which promotes filteration of water and all non-colloidal constituents of plasma that is uric acid, salts, glucose, amino acids. The fluid filtered passes downwards in the convoluted tubules. The epithelium of the tubules reabsorbs. fluid of the same composition as normal blood plasma without its colloidal constituents absorbing glucose and amino acids while excretory materials such as urea, uric acid abnormal salts are not reabsorbed along with acid radicals. The rate of this glomerular filteration depends on the difference of pressure but the blood and interior of Bowman's Capsule. Besides circulation in the kidneys influenced by influence of digestion and assimilation in the urine. Gastric digestion tends to make the urine alkaline as quantity of acid is withdrawn from blood. This is increased when digestion begins, water and alkaline salts enter the blood which increase the alkalinity of urine. Volume of blood rises and renal secretion is increased, finally metabolic products from liver, lungs etc. also enter the blood and appear in the urine. After digestion water escapes with alkaline salts, excess of urea, uric acid is excreted and after three hours of digestion it again becomes acid. Besides kidneys produced internal secretion which diminishes metabolic waste matter and the production of urea. Ayurveda knew the law of circulation as mentioned in the above Shlokas. Besides Ayurveda science also had the knowledge to some extent about bacteria.

रक्त वाहि शिरा स्थान रक्त जा जन्त वो अठावः ।
अपाद वृत्तास्तां ब्राश्व सौस्म्याल केचित दर्शनः ॥

Some bacteria spread in the body through blood.. The bacteria have no legs of any kind, they are circular and reddish looking. Some are so minute that they are invisible to the eyes.

गद निग्रह कृषि रोगा धिकार सुचुता चार्य Says:
कृमीन्बहु विधा कारान्करोति विविधाश्रयान् ।

Bacteria are of various kinds and they live in different parts for example poisonous fevers are described to be due to the bites of mosquitoes.

भूता भिषं गोत्यम् वुवेत विषय ज्वरम । (वाग्भर Says) अशुचीत नाक्रमेत-
Do not walk over the diet.

In Ayurveda certain medicines are described to have antiseptic properties such as sun-light (सुर्यप्रकाश), fire (अग्नि) pure air (हवा), sulphur (गंधक), mercur perchloride (रसकपुर) and black lay. Besides the blood vessel Ayurveda mentions of system of vessels which carry Ras (रस), Biv juices formed out of food during the processes of digestion in the intestines and Ras (रस) from the tissues. This is probably the lymphatic system mentioned in the Western science of medicine as follows:

The lymphatic vessels in the small intestines are called lacteals and they contain a milky white fluid the chyle. In most of the tissues of the body there are also minute spaces and channels which contains lymph. Ras (रस) formed out transudation of fluid Ras (रक्तरस) from capillaries and acted upon by tissue changes and moved on in lymphatic. These lymphatic vessels are exceedingly delicate. They present a beaded appearance. They are fitted in all parts of the body except nonvascular structures such as cartilage, nails, cuticle and hair. They are arranged into superficial and deep set. Superficial lymphatics accompany the superficial veins and form the deep lymphatic vessels at certain parts. In the interior of the body they lie in the submucus areolar tissue throughout the whole length of the digestive, respiratory and genito-urinary tracts and in the sub-serous tissue of the thoracic and abdominal walls. From the net works of lymphatics in the tissues small vessels converge, which pass to a gland close by or enter into larger lymphatic vessels, deep lymphatics follow deep vessels. Thoracic duct conveys the chyle and greater part of lymph of the body into the blood into the left sub-clavian vein while the right thoracic duct which takes the lymph from the right side of the head, neck, thoracic wall, right upper extremity, right lung; right side of the heart; opens into right subclavian vein and thus the lymph enters the circulation.

Chapter VI

Composition of Body

Now according to the Western science this body consists of organic and inorganic elements, carbon, oxygen, hydrogen, nitrogen, iron, calcium, magnesium, sulphur, potassium, phosphorous, sodium, flourine, chlorine and silica.

In Ayurveda this body is composed of animal (प्राणिज) and earthy matters (पार्थिव) and both these are made of 5 elements (पृथ्वी, आप, तेज, वायु, आणि आकाश) Earth (पृथ्वी) contains calcium, sodium, phosphorous, sulphur, magnesia, potassium, silica, chlorine, flourine, iron and other things.

Water (आप) contains hydrogen and oxygen.

Tej (तेज) contains heat and energy.

Ait (वायु) contains oxygen, nitrogen and carbon etc.

Sky (आकाश) etherial space.

It will be seen, there is no difference as regards the origin of the body. Western science says that this body is composed of cells. Ayurveda says the same.

शरीरा वय वास्तु परमाणु भेदे ना परि संख्येया ।
भवन्ति अति वहुत्वादति अति सौक्ष्म्यवाद तीद्रियत्वाञ्च ॥
चरक शारीर स्थान अयाध्या 7 ।

By the division of cells, the limbs are formed and these cells are very minute and invisible. Ayurveda further says that this body which is made of innumerable invisible cells and which is developed from the original seed cell;

Beej Paramanu (बीज परिमाणु) is invested with and which the properties of protoplasm is fed and developed by a process of metabolism. (दानोपदान क्रिया) .

Can Western science dis prove this?

As in Western science are described various systems such as nervous, digestive, circulatory, urinary systems etc.

In the same way Ayurveda describes three systems Vat, Pitt and Kuff (वात, पित्त और कफ).

The functions of Vat, Pitt and Kuff have already been described. Functions of Vat to give in brief are respiration and micturition to keep circulation of blood in order, deglutition, speech, muscular activity, remembrance sneezing, yawning, etc. Functions at Pitt hunger, thirst, digestion, body heat, production of body juices for digestion, vision etc. Functions of Kuff regulation of cohesive force and regulation of water in the system to keep the body united and proportionate; to and keep fluid in the joints. It appears therefore.

Vat (वात) as mentioned in the Ayurveda carries on the functions of central and symphathetic nervous systems.

Pitt (पित्त) carries on the process of metabolism and digestion and assimilations.

Kuff (कफ) has the function of control of oxidation and production of fluid for the protection of ogans such an fluid in the pleura. Peritoneum and joints.

Ayurveda says Vat is the principal factor which regulate, all the systems in the body and it divides Vat into प्राण, अपान, व्यान, उदान और समान.

For example Pran vayu (प्राण वायु) carries on respiration.

Wyan vayu (व्यान वायु) gives oxygen (vishnoo-padamrut) to the tissues.

Pitt (पित्त) is also divided into digestive (पाचक) रंजक, साधक, भ्राजक और आलोचक :—

Its functions are to digest and produce body cells to be utilized for the body. These functions may be called according to Western science production of enzymes during digestion.

Kuff (कफ़) is also divided into five; क्लेदक, अवलंबक, बोधक, तर्पक और अश्लेषक.

Its functions are to regulate body heat, to lubricate the joints, to keep the parts such as pleura, peritoneum etc. moist for the protection of the organs underneath.

When these, Pitt and Kuff are working in order, they are called Dhatu (धातु)) and when in disorder they are called Dosh (दोष).

This diseases are called : 3/4 वात रोग, पित्त रोग, कफ़ रोग या वात पित्त रोग, कफ़ पित्त रोग, वात पित्त कफ रोग.

When two are in excess it is called Dwidosh (द्विदोष) and three (त्रिदोष).

हृदोरसा निश्चरति तम्मा देवच सर्वशः ।
शिराभिः हृदयं चेती तस्मा तत्प्रभवाः शिराः ॥
(भेड संहितादश मूलियाध्याय)

Blood goes out of the heart to all parts and returns again through veins.

शिराधमन्यो; नाभिस्थाः सर्वं व्याप्य स्थितास्तनुम् ।
पुष्णन्ति चानिश वायो; संयो गात्सर्व धातुभिः ॥
प्रथम खंड अध्याय 5 । शार्ङ्गधर

Veins and arteries are all over the body. They are always night and day acting and support the body.

नाभिस्थः प्राण पवनः स्पृष्यवा हृत्कमलांतरम् ।
कंठा घ्दर्विनिर्याति पातुं विष्णु पदामृतम् ॥
पीत्वा चांबर पीसूषं पुनरायाति वेगतः ।
प्रीणायन् देहमखिलं जीवंच जठरा नलमू ॥
प्रथम खंड अध्याय 5 । शार्ङ्गधर

Vayu (धातु) from near the navel forces the air from the lungs outside the throat and it again takes Vishnoo-Padamrut i.e. oxygen and throwing out vitiated matter it comes again in the lungs and this way keeps the body in pleasant condition. Blood supplies all necessary things to the tissues and unnecessary parts are taken out through urine, faeces etc.

This is called metabolism (दानोपदाम क्रिया) out of this seven dhatus are formed. Health of the body depends on proper and regular metabolism and that action depends on food, air, water, exercise and digestion. Ayurveda divides the food into two parts organic and inorganic.

In Organic—All kinds of meat and vegetables are included. Animal food consists of (अन्नि, जल, पृथ्वी, वायु और आकाश). While vegetable food is full of sour, bitter, saltish, acid and sweet juices.

In Inorganic food there is water, salt, calcium salts and it consists of (अग्नि और जल).

Animal food increases blood and other Sapta Dhatu (सप्ता धातु) and creates energy, strength and appetite. Flesh increases flesh. Water is considered very valuable. Common salt is digestive and increases the digestive juices. It is not given in cases of Dropsy. Ayurveda considers mixed diet to be the best for health. Ayurved lays great stress on (ब्रह्मचर्य)) i.e. to lead a celebate life more or less. This is necessary for health and to produce good progeny.

As regards the excretion Ayurveda says that some are solid such as faeces, some are semi-solid such as sputum and some are liquid such as urine and perspiration and some are gaseous such as out-going breath, and wind from the rectum etc.

Chapter VII

Diseases from वाग्भट अध्याय 2 नदान and चिकित्सा स्थान अ. 3

Fevers (ज्वर) they are of eight kinds बात ज्वर, पित्त ज्वर, कफ ज्वर, वात पित्त ज्वर.

They are due to excess of दोष in वात, पित्त and Kuff (कफ़). Certain symptoms are malaise, feeling out of sorts, pains in the limbs, headache, rise of temperature, bad taste in the mouth and thirst etc. In Pitt fever there is vomiting, high temperature, bad taste in the mouth, acid eructations, some eruptions, symptoms of indigestion and foul breath.

In Kuff fever—Low temperature, cough, breathlessness, vomiting, sweet-taste in the mouth etc.

In Vat-Pitt fever—Combination of symptoms given above.

In Vat-Pitt-Kuff fever—there is combination of symptoms of all three but this is accompanied by alternate sensation of cold and heat, sleeplessness, profuse perspiration, pains in the joints, palpitation, diarhoea in some cases, stickiness in the mouth etc. Fevers due to burns, injuries are due to inflammation and are attended with symptoms of local inflammation. In nervous fever there is a good deal of headache with other general symptoms. Seasonal fevers are due to climatic conditions and they resemble more or less Vat-Pitt-Kuff fevers.

Eruptive fevers such as small-pox, measles, chicken-pox etc, show exaggerated symptoms of fever noticed in Vat, Pitt and Kuff type and are accompanied with characteristic eruptions. Poisonous fevers are typhoid (विषम), malarial and septiceamic.

Typhoid fevers are classed as fourteen days, eighteen days and 22 days fever and they last sometimes many days.

Malarial fevers are classed as one, three and four days fevers. They are more or less called as (वातकफात्मक) fevers. They are more or less accompanied with severe pains in back, severe headache and profuse perspiration.

Remittent fevers (संतत्र) (एकसा) are classed as seven days, ten days and twelve days fevers. They arise from (दोष) dosh in वात्, पित्त and कफ.

General treatment—Fasting or very light food emetics or purgatives as the symptoms of Vat, Pitt and Kuff are in excess. Luke-warm water to drink to allay thirst, when digestive symptoms are prominent, decoction of (नागर मोथा,) Nagar motha, (चंदन वाला) Chandan wala and (पित्त पापला) Pittpapala should be given three times a day to produce perspiration. Diet— (लाहि) Dalia of grain lightly boiled with little rock-salt (सैंधण मीढें) may be given. If there be vomitting little ginger and honey. Constipation is treated with a decoction of (पिपलमुल), Piplemul, (मनुका) (dried grapes), Awla (आंवला) and ginger and cocum. These may be given in first three or four days. In eruptive fevers such as small-pox, measles, etc., only symptomate treatment is followed. In Vat-Juwar (fever) decoction of (गुलवेल) Gulwel ginger and (पिपलमुंल) Pilemul one oz, three times a day. Pitta-jwar (fever) decoction of Indrajav and Nagarmotha (इन्द्रजव और नागरमोथा)

one ounce thrice daily. Kuff-fever (कफ ज्वर) (हिरड्या) Hirda, (पिंपलमुल) Piplemul and गुलवेल Gulwel ounce of decoction three times a day.

Kuff wat fevers (कफ वात ज्वर) decoction (वखंड) Wekhand (पहाड़ मुल) Pahadmul and (गुलवेल) Gulwel one ounce thrice.

In Sannipat (सीन्नपात) fevers infusion of (रिंगणीमुळ), Ringnimul, (देवदार) Dewdar, (हल्दी) Haldi, (नागरमोथा) Nagarmotha and (त्रिफला) Tiphala one ounce three or four times a day. In fevers accompanied with cold (Malarial) Infusion of Neem leaves, (गुलवेल) Gulwel and (रिंगणी) Ringni one ounce 3 or 4 times a day. Besides boiled cow's milk, whey, soups of different kinds can also be given to keep the strength, Western science classifies fevers as follows:

Specific fevers: Small-pox, measles, chicken-pox etc.

Inflammatory fevers:—Pneumonia, Pleurisy etc.

Fevers due to local disease: Indigestion, Extravasation, Never-debility, fright etc.

Fevers due to injury:

Causes of fever are due to metabolic changes in the tissues which increase the heat production or dimunition of heat, loss regulated normally by heat regulating centre in the corpus-striatum. General treatment: Diet should be light, digestible and nutritious. Antipyretic drugs to reduce the temperature such as Quinine, Phenatecin and diphoretics etc.

Ayurveda says that fevers are due to excess of Vat, Pitt and Kuff in the system or to their disordered action which gives rises to excessive heat and which is not eliminated through the organs or pores of the skin. This excess of production of heat is due to poisons circulating in the body system which tend to derange or exaggerate the normal functions of the principal factors mentioned above.

Fevers arising purely from derangement of nervous system as seen in cases of cerebral haemorrhage, passage of gall stones and other neurotic fevers can be compared to fevers in Ayurveda arising from *Vat* alone.

Specific-fevers: Which are due to the bacterial toxins acting on the heat centre such as typhus, scarletina, measles etc. are according to Ayurveda due to excess of *Pitt* production in the system due to toxins.

Fevers in cases like Consumption are probably due to Rakt, Pitt and Kuff. *Symptoms:*—Acid eructations, burning sensation in the mouth, vomiting, cough, foulbreath.

Cough is divided to वातकास, पित्तकास, कफ़कास, और क्षतकास.

Vatkas (वातकास) It is dry and constant sensation of coughing with scanty expectoration.

Pittkas. पित्तकास acid and bitter taste in the mouth slight Jaundice, vomiting, acid eructations with some expectoration.

Kuffkas. (कफकास)—It is accompanied with thick sticky white expectorations.

Kshaya and Kshayakas (क्षय और क्षयकास)—It is accompanied with purulent, foul smelling, yellowish or red expectoration.

Treatment—Fasting or light food or mild purgative.

To promote vomitting गेलफल (gelphal) may be given in little honey or milk. This is followed by one ounce of infusion of शतावरी (Shatawary) अडुलसा (Adulsa) काकोली (Kakoli) ज्येष्टमध (Jeshtamadh) (Mulethe) three times a day.

Bacterial toxins and local inflammations are according to Ayurveda due to excess of Kuff production in the system due to bacterial and other inflammatory products acting on that force and deranging it and mixed types of fevers are due to derangement of either of two factors.

Breathlessness (श्वास), Asthma (दमा) and Hiccough (उचकी).

This breathlessness is classed as शुद्, Kshudra-light, तमक, Tamak-severe छिन्न, Chinna-Broken महान, Mahan-severe उर्ध्व Urdwa-Rising.

These are the different stages of Asthma.

Slight breathlessness goes under the name of क्षुद्र श्वास Kshurdra swas.

It is cured gradually without any medicine on improvement of general health.

तमक श्वास Tamak swas—Accompanied by cough and cold, thirst and patient feels better after little expectoration.

छिन्न श्वास—Chinna swas is accompanied with perspiration, fainting, digestive disorders such as constipation, interrupted breathing and dryness in the mouth.

महान श्वास—Mahan swas all the symptoms of छिन्नश्वास are exaggerated.

उर्ध्व श्वास—Urdhwa swas this is accompanied with great difficulty in breathing.

Hiccoughs are of five kinds:

1. Due to disorders of digestion.
2. This originates by some irritation in the stomach and is increased by some work and decreased after food.

This is called शुद्र kshudra.

यमला—Yamala this begins about two hours after food and is accompanied with vomiting and great thirst.

महती—Mahati it is accompanied with exaggeration of above palpitation, great dryness in the mouth and distension of abdomen.

गंभीरा—Gambhira it shows all the symptoms of Mahati (महती) but it is accompanied with yawning, pains in the head and stomach and it is very frequent and louder.

Treatment for Asthma (दमा)
Dried grapes four tolas.
Dashamul (दशमूल) two tolas.
Shatawary (शतावरी) two tolas.
Kulith (कुलीथ) Kulith a sort of grain—20 tolas.
Ber (बेर) ... ... 20 tolas.
Java (जब) ... ... 20 tolas.
Water ... ... 3 pints.

One ounce of decoction should be given 3 times a day or a powder made out of:

वायबिडंग... ... one tola
Wawbiding
Ginger ... do —
रास्ना ... do —
Rasna
Asafoetidia (हिंग) 1/2 tola
Rock salt (सेंधानमक) do —
Bharang mul (भांरगमूल) do —
Javakhat (जवखाट) do —

10 grains of this powder may be given in the case of adult three times with little of water.

Constipation is to be treated with a mild purgative such as castor oil and food should be very light. In severe cases goats fat in little honey, sugar and ghee in small quantity is beneficial. When there is blood in expectoration:

Punarnava	...	...	...	One tola
Sugar	...	...	...	One tola
Old rice grain	...	...	...	Four toals
Mahuwa	...	...	...	One tola
Mulethi	...	...	...	One tola

Ten grains of this in little of milk is also beneficial. Leaves of हल्दी (Haldi), एरंडमूल (Erandmul) dried grapes मनशील (Mansil), देवदार (Dewdar), और जटामांसी (Jatamansi) should be powdered and spread on the cloth and mixed with a little of Gugul (गुगुल) and set on fire and should be inhaled.

Treatment of hiccough as follows:

Mild purgatives, and emetics, light food and fomentation over the stomach.

Garlic	...	...	One	Tola
पिपली (Pimpli)	...	...	,,	,,
काला नमक (Black salt)	...		,,	,,
आंवला (Awla)	...	...	,,	,,
Asafoetida	..	...	Half	,,
हर्र (Harrar)	...	...	,,	,,
Rock salt	...	...	,,	,,

Ten grains of this to an adult may be given.

Consumption राज यक्ष्मा.

This disease is accompanied by chronic cough, loss of appetite, wasting, and loss of sleep, foul breath owing to disorder in Vat, Pitt and Kuff. Food juices are not properly formed and assimilated. Fever comes daily or on certain days with night sweats. Expectoration in muc-purulent and pain in the head and chest, haemoptysis and breathlessness and inability to digest and later on diarrhoea and change in the voice.

Treatment—Soups and meat and goats milk and ghee and pure air. Mutton soup mixed with decoction of पिंपली (Pipeli), यव (Yow), डालिंब (Dalimb), Pomogranate, आंवला (Awla) is beneficial. An infusion of रास्ना चिकना (Rasna-chikna), गोखरू (Gokhru), सालवण (Salwan), घटोली (Ghatoli) and पिंपळी (Pipepli) should be taken 3 times a day.

Bansh-lochan	8 tolas
Cinnamon	1 tolas
Cardamoms	2 tolas
Pipeli	4 tolas
Sugar	16 tolas

60 grains of this may be taken three times a day.

Vomiting (बांती) are of five kinds due to disorders of Vat, Pitt and Kuff in the stomach.

Treatment—Mild purgative and light food or fasting. In vomiting due to Pitt—An initial emetic should be given to clean out the stomach and an infusion of Pipeli and Dhane (पिपली धने) an ounce every fourth hour also does good. In (बांती) vomiting due to Kuff (कफ), an initial emetic is also good. An infusion of Jav (जव) Barley water mixed with lemon-juice acts well.

Heart Diseases

Their symptoms are—thirst, paleness, fainting, vomiting and loss of sleep. In heart disease due to Vat (वात) headache and palpitation and loss of appetite and sleeplessness and pain over the heart.

When due to Pitt (पित्त) Acid eructations, paleness, vomiting and fever.

When due to Kuff (कफ) cough, loss of appetite, fever and bad taste in the mouth. In (सन्निपातिक हृदरोग) (Sannipaterhoudrog). All the symptoms are combined.

In (कृमि जन्य) Krumi-janya (septic) disease there is constant palpilation over the heart region, breathlessness and vomiting and cough thrist (तृष्णा). This is due to excess of Vayu and Pitt (वायु and पित्त). It is also due to bloodlessness.

In thirst due to Vat (वात) there is headache, giddiness and loss of appetite and when due to Pitt it is accompanied with fever and bad taste in the mouth.

In heart disease—Ayurveda prescribes all sorts of meat juices and milk.

In heart disease due to Pitt (पित्त) grape and sugarcane juice and rest,

In heart disease due to Kuff (कफ) an infusion of (हिरडा) Hirda-harra ginger and (कायफळ) Kayphal three times a day is recommended. In thirst honey and water.

When due to Vat (वात) Gul (गुळ) and curd twice a day and when to Pitt (पित्त) an infusion of ज्येस्टमध (Jeshtamadh-Mulethi).

In thirst due to excess of alcohol acid drinks such as lemon juice and water is useful and when due to indigestion a little water and Gul (गुळ) should be taken after food and if that does not allay any emetic may be taken. In thirst due to debility—mutton soup.

Ayurveda says almost all the lung affections such as Bronchitis, Asthma, Consumption and Pneumonia etc. are due to excess of Kuff (कफ). When this is in lungs, this blocks the porous openings in the lungs and acts on Vat (वात) that is the power by which expiration and inspiration of the lungs are effected. This indirectly acts on the heart through (रसास) Rasas in the blood and causes symptoms of (हृद्रोग) heart diseases.

Western science defines the diseases of the lungs as (1) various inflammations of bronchi, Asthma, and their obstruction and its effects on the lungs causing a loss of elasticity...from obstruction and weakening and subsequent atrophy and destruction of Lung tissue contained in the alveolar septa (Emphysema.)

Exudation of serous fluid in the lungs causing oedema of the lungs.

Inflammation of the substance of the lungs is called Pneumonia due to various organisms. When local involving a small bronchi and a part of lung it is called Broncho-Pneumonia leading in some cases to gangrine.

Tubercle of the lung: That is invasion of tubercle bacilli and the formation of tubercles in the lung tissue as the result of irritation of the bacilli. The occurrence of Pneumonic processes in connection with tubercles, the consolidation of the lung around them and subsequent of those areas in to cavities and their suppuration and discharge by expectoration and general constitutional disturbance in consequence.

Spasmodic bronchial condition of the smaller destruction tubes causing dyspnoea...such sudden attacks subsiding after a time and recurring at irregular intervals is called Asthma.

In Ayurveda all these diseases attributes to derangement of Kuff **(कफ)** and consequent vitiation of Vat **(वात)**. Ayurveda did not know the minute anatomy of long tissue but the symptoms of those diseases as described in it are more or less accurate.

Heart Diseases: Ayurveda describes these to be of 5 kinds—when due to derangement of Vat **(वात)** it causes precordical pain, palpitation, nervine temper and paleness and yellowness of skin, breathlessness and loss of sleep.

Symptoms of other heart diseases are already given.

This description is very inaccurate though symptoms tally to some extent according to Western science. It classifies the diseases as follows:—

1. Diseases arising from heart muscle such as hypertrophy dilatation and hypertrophy and dilatation, inflammation and fatty degeneration.

2. Diseases arising from the defects in the endocardium—such as endocarditis whether malignant or simple and diseases of the valves such as Aortic and mitral regurgitation etc.

3. Functional diseases of the heart such as Tachy cardia Auricular fibrilation etc.

4. Nervine...diseases such as Angina-pectoris etc.

5. Discases of pericardium such as pericardities etc.

No mentnion is made in Ayurveda about Aneurism and mediastinal new growths.

Diseases of the blood vessels Phlebites thrombosis and Cinbolism vasomotor disorders such as excessive pulsation or throbbing of arteries are not mentioned.

Symptoms of heart disease as given in Ayurveda are not accurate and character of the pulse has not been described nor Ayurveda knew anything about the murmurs, and effects of heart diseases on different organs. Although Ayurveda knew that the heart contracts and dilates they did not know the sounds of the hearts nor their exact position. They did not know the exact area occupied by the heart in the body.

They had some knowledge about the pulse as they constantly felt it at the wrist, but Ayurveda only knew that it as fast, slow, irregular or small. Ayurveda does not describe the rate of the pulse and rhythm, volume of the pulse and its hardness. They did not know venous pulsation. As the knowledge about the heart and arteries was little the treatment in Ayurveda about these diseases is not satisfactory.

Decoction of (सेंधव) Saindhawa, (जवखार) Jawakhar, (वेखंड) Wekhand, (जिरे) Jire, (सुंठ) Sunth, (देवदार) Dewdar, (ओंवा) Owa, (महालुंग) Mahalulung, (हिरडे) Hirde four tolas of each in three parts of water. One ounce of this is to be taken twice a day, but these medicines are more or less stomachic tonic and aperient. Western science deals with various detailed treatment of heart diseases and their symptoms.

1. Rest, to take off all possible strain from the heart.
2. Relief of circulation by purgative and diruetics and diaphretics and venesection.
3. Light and easily digestible diet.
4. By drugs to strengthen the heart muscle and its beat.
5. Symptomatic treatment as the symptoms arise.

Chapter VIII

Diseases from Digestive Troubles

They are (अर्श) Arsh Piles, (अतिसार) Atisar, (ग्रहणी) Grahani, and (गुल्म) Gulma.

(अर्श) Arsh—Dry piles i.e. those which do not bleed.

They arise from vitiated blood and excess of Pitt giving rise to indigestion, straining friction around the anus and debility due to diarrhoea, heart and liver diseases. They cause symptoms of indigestion such as vomiting, constipation, acid eructations and gurgling in the abdomen, pains in the head, stomach and debility.

Those that are due to Vat are reddish looking, hard, curved, round or pedunculated, cause good deal of staining and pain at the time of defaecation and debility and afterwards enlargement of liver and spleen and dropsy.

Those that are due to Pitt. They are yellowish or blackish in colour, soft and loose. They are narrow at the base and cause semi-liquid motions mixed with blood.

Those that are due to Kuff are not so painful. They are superficial sticky and cause itching sensation in and around anus and do not bleed.

Those that arise from (सान्निपती) Sannipati—They are red, very painful, inflamed and bleed.

Treatment.—Mild purgatives, light diet, little juice of (मदार) Madar, (निवडुंग) Nivdung, (कडु दुर्वाचा पाला) Kadu durvacha pala. करंज (Karanj) seeds well pounded should be applied over the piles.

Enema once a day. (सेंधव) Saidhav, grs. X. (पादेलोन) Padelon, grs. X, (डिबलोन) Bidlon, grs. Ginger grs. X and as (अमलवेतस) Amlawatus grs. I. asafoetida grs. II, should be taken once a day in hot water.

(अतिसार)–(Atisar) diarrhoea these are of six kinds. It arises from eating bad food, worms, and other digestive troubles. Faeces are semi-liquid, contain mueus and are frequent. These are the symptoms of वातातिसार.

In पितातिसार–(Pittatisar) stools are yellow, reddish or greenish looking and contains blood, foul smelling and frequent and are accompanied with good deal of pain.

कफातिसार–(Kufatisar) stools are more or less white, sticky contain undigested matter and cause straining.

त्रिदोशत्मक अतिसार–(Tridoshatmak Atisar) stools are very liquid, like water and contains very little faecal matter.

आमातिसार– (Amatisar) stools are very foul smelling and are painful.

Treatment–Fasting or very light food and one ounce of decoction of the following twice a day.

ओवा (Owa) Ani seeds zi. पिंपळी (Pipeli) zi. Ginger zi. Bekhand zii, धने (Dhane) zi and हिरडे दल Hirde dal zii. Water three pints or milk 8 ounces; water 24 ounces Nagarmotha 20 dramchs.

Should be boiled and strained and milk taken once a day. Jambuls, डालिंब, चुका, कमलाचा कांदा Dalimb, Chuka, Kamalke beej, one ounce each in 20 ounces of water and boiled and strained.

ग्रहणी – Grahani causes headache, fever, burning sensation in the mouth, and distension of stomach.

वात ग्रहणी–Vat Grahani causes frequent motions, stools are semi-solid foul smelling and painful.

पित्त ग्रहणी–(Pitt grahani) causes yellow or greenish stools, acid eructations and thirst.

कफ ग्रहणी–(Kuff Grahani) causes vomiting, stickiness in the mouth, sweet eructations, stools contain good deal of mucus.

त्रिदोष ग्रहनी–(Tridosh Grahani) stools are painful, semi solid or liquid yellowish or greenish and very foul smelling.

Treatment—Light and digestive food, soups, whey old and light rice, (डालिंब) Dalimb honey and goat's milk

हिरडा	Hirda	4	Dr. mchs
जिरे	Geere	1	-do-
पादेलोन	Padalon	2	-do-
मिरे	Mire	1	-do-
बिडलोन	Bidlon	1	-do-

To be powdered—10 grains of this to be taken twice a day. Enema or emetic as required.

गुलम – (Gulma) causes colic and distension of the stomach and intestines.

वात गुलम–(Vat gulma) causes headache, enlarged spleen, gurgling in the intestines, constipation, thirst.

पित्त गुलम–(Pitt gulma) – Acid eructation, diarrhoea, perspiration and pain.

कफ गुलम (Kuff Gulma) – Causes distension of stomach, cold and loss of appetite.

सन्निपात गुलम (Sannipati Gulma) – Colic is very severe accompanied with fever.

रक्त गुलम (Rakat Gulma) – This only occurs among women, which causes severe pain in the uterus, diarrhoea, thirst and fever.

Treatment. Enema

Rock salt one tola,

Ajmoda (अजमोदा) two tolas,

Owa (ओवा) Anisi three tolas,

Pipli (पिंपली) four tolas,

Ginger (सुंठ) five tolas.

To be powdered and 30 grains to be taken twice a day before food.

Asafoetida—one tola.

Rock salt—three tolas,

Castor oil—nine tolas,

Garlic juice—one tola,

30 drops to be taken twice a day.

When there is haemorrhage from the womb in case of women, little Gur (गुल) and Jawakhar should be put at the mouth of the womb and fomentations.

अजीर्ण (Ajeern) Indigestion.

This is due to drinking large quantity of water. Irregular time for food and sleep, bad quality of food.

अग्निमांदय, अलस्य आणि विषुचिका. (Agnimandya, Alasya and Wishuchika).

They are also due to digestive troubles due to derangement in Pitt.

Treatment—Soups of all kinds, old moong or rice stomachics such as Garlic, Ginger, Chandbel chuka, Jawkhar, Paperkhar, Asafoetida, when indigestion becomes acute causing pain in the stomach and eructations and distension it is called Alas and when all the limbs become painful with good deal of distension of the abdomen it is called Wishuchika (विषुचिका). Western science classifies the diseases of the digestive system into diseases of stomach arising from inflammation of mucus membrane, such as gatritis, ulcers, cancer, etc., obstruction (stenosis) and functional disorder giving rise to indigestion and atony. Ayurveda only describes one disease called Ajeerna (अजीर्ण). Ayurveda had knowledge of secretions of the glands of the stomach but it did not know its exact anatomy and topography, nor the secretion of free hydrochloric acid nor its motor power of the muscle. Hence all diseases of the stomach which caused inflammation such as gastritis, ulcer, cancer etc. went under the name of Wanti (वांती) stenosis or dilatation of stomach it did not notice.

Under diseases of intestines are mentioned (अतिसार) Atisar (ग्रहणी) Grahni, (गुलम) Gulma. They are diarrhoea, cuteritis and various kinds of tumours in connection with intestines and constipation and intestinal colic. Ayurveda did not know the diseases arising from alimentary taximia nor intestinal stasis nor the actions of specific baclli in the intestinal tract and skin eruptions depending upon gastro-intestinal irritation. The description of diarrhoea in Ayurveda is very imcomplete, Western science divides it into Acute and chronic diarrhoea, choleric in which the stools are profuse and watery or rice water-coloured, dysenteric in which mucus and blood is present, lienteric in which there are undigested food particles. Bilious in which the stools are deeply stained with bile and its derivatives and colliquative when it gets profuse and exhausting. Enteritis is divided into acute and chronic arising from irritation of mucus membrane due to unsuitable food and certain poisons such as food poisoning (Ptomain poisoning).

Sprue is chronic catarrhal enteritis which occurs in the tropics. Again enteritis may be diptheretic or phlegmonous. There is no mention of appendicitis and diseases caused by tubercle or new growths or intestinal obstructions. Intussuception.

Constipation is the retention of faeces for longer than the normal period of 24 hours. The defect in the final process of defaecation i.e. in the passge of faeces into the rectum and the final evacuation is the cause of habitual constipation. The constant repression of the desire and disregard of sensation are common causes of constipation. It is also due to weakness of the voluntary muscles which compress the abdominal contents. Dyspepsia is the term used to indicate any modification of the process of digestion resulting imperfect solution of food by the gatric secretions, delayed transmission, flatulence, the excessive formation of flatus associated with nausea are common symptoms of dyspepsia.

Dyspepsia is divided into flatulent dyspepsia, acid dyspepsia, atonic dyspepsia, and nervous kind. Hyperchlorhydria, there is more or less buring pain lasting for 2 or 3 hours after food accompanied with acid eructations. These pains diminish by foods richer in proteins.

Haemorrhcids are due to anything that tends to congestion of the portal system such as heart and liver diseases and are also due to anything determining local congestion of the part such as habitual constipation, straining at stools, distended colon etc.

External Piles—are soft globular pinkish blue swellings. Ayurveda calls these due to excess of Kuff.

Internal Piles—may be either slightly raised, flat or oblong elevations or distinctly globular or pedunculated. They originate owing to increase of Pitt according to Ayurveda. They begin to bleed when the mucus membrane covering them is congested and becomes very painful when it is inflamed. In some cases these piles are firm and fleshy and are of a reddish brown colour and they do not bleed. Sometimes these both external and internal become inflamed and slough. The description given as regards the symptoms of the piles and the varities resemble more or less to the description given in medical books of Western science and also its treatment to some extent.

जलोदर (Jalodar)—Ascitis.

This disease begins with indigestion and to derangement in Vat and Kuff.

Symptoms Loss of appetite, burning sensation in the throat breathlessness, distension, slight oedema of the feet, visible veins on the abdomen, pains in the back and loins and abdomen. They are of eight kinds:

वातोदर (Vatoder)-symptoms—coldness in the hands and feet and swelling, pains in the joints, heaviness in the lower part of abdomen and its distension and visible veins on it and feeling of water movement in the abdomen on tapping.

पित्तोदर (Pittoder)-symptoms—fever, diarrhoea, jaundice, greenish tinge on the abdomen, visible veins and sensation of water in the abdomen.

कफोदर (Kafoder)– Swelling of the feet, distension of abdomen, breathlessness, cough, paleness of the skin, pale veins on the abdomen.

सन्निपातोदर (Sannipatoder)– All the symptons given above are exaggerated.

पिलहोदर (Pilhoder)–Here there is distinct enlargement of spleen in abdomen.

वद्धोदर (Vadhoder)–This occurs in some cases of obstinate constipation or obstruction of intestines.

क्षतोदर (Shatoder)–This occurs in case of rupture of intestines.

जलोदर (Jaloder)–It is accompanied with breathlessness and extensive distension of abdomen, covered with veins and gives sensation of fluid moving on tapping.

Treatment: Light and easily digestible food; Cow's or camel's milk, purgatives and diuretics and diaphoretic drugs. Whey from cow's milk जव, बोरे व कुलिथ (Jav, Bore; Kulith) Decoction of these three in equal quantities is said to be useful. In later stages when the abdomen is very much distended, tapping and drawing off the fluid. When mixed with little, पिंपली (Pipeli) and rock salt is useful, in वातोदर (Vatoder) little मिरे (Mire) and sugar, in पित्तोदर (Pittoder) anisi and rock salt. जिरे (Jeere) in कफोदर (Kafoder), जवखार (Jawakhar) and Rock Salt, is सन्निपातोदर (Sannipatoder) with honey बेखंड (Bekhand), Ginger and Salt, in जलोदर (Jaloder) due to enlarged spleen. Ascitis according to Western science is the presence of serious fluid in the peritoneal cavity arising from obstruction in the portal circulation, either in the trunk of portal vein or in its branches (2) as the result of the diseases of peritoneum (3) as a part of the general dropsy of kidney disease. Ayurveda does not describe the dull percussion note caused by the fluid nor the signs of fluctuation and the method of displacement.

पित्तोदर (Pithodar) is due to inflammation of kidneys and वातोदर (Vatodar) to heart diseases and कफोदर (Kafodar) to liver diseases and obstruction in portal circulation. In heart disease it begins in feet and ankles and gradually extends up to the legs but even when it is very extensive it is generally confined to the lower extremities and lower half of the Trunk leaving face, chest, arms, and hands free. In cases due to portal obstruction the fluid first begins to accumulate in the abdomen.

It becomes generally tense and globular, later on the walls of the abdomen become distended and as the patient moves, the fluid graviates in flanks, and the abdomen becomes proportionately enlarged which gives a dull note to the percussion. As the fiuid increases the dullness encroaches from the sides to the centre and at length only a limited area becomes resonant occasionally the abdomen is entirely dull. When the abdomen becomes tense, veins become visible over the surface.

In renal dropsy it involves the whole surface of the body. The first change appears in the puffiness of the eye-lids when the patient rises in the morning. This subsides in the course of the day, at night time there is slight oedema of the ankles. Oedema generally is in the most depended parts. In more advanced cases the face becomes full and rounded and the eye lids are distended, limbs become enlarged and shapeless, the trunk is enlarged. When this dropsy becomes general it is called Anasarka. With this general dropsy there is also a effusion in all cavities.

पांडूरोज (Pandurog) Anaemea from वाग्भट Vagbhata They are due to Vat, Pitt and Kuff and called वात जन्य (Vat janya), पित्तजन्य (Pitta janya), कफजन्य (Kuff janya), आणि सन्निपात जन्य (Sannipat janya).

Symptoms: General debility, breathlessness, palpitation, dryness of the skin, yellowish urine.

वात पांडूरोग (Vat Pandurog): General pains all over the body, dark tinge round the eyes and nails. When due to Pitt there is fever and yellowish tinge of the skin, perspiration, diarrhoea and acid eructations and when due to Kuff there is paleness and white tinge on the skin accompanied with cough and vomiting. When due to सन्निपात (Sannipat) all these symptoms are exaggerated.

Treatment: Decoction of अडूलसा (Adulsa), गुलबेल (Gulbel), त्रिफला (Trifala), कटुकी (Katuki), कडु किरायत व (Kadu kirayat), कडूनिंब (Kadunimb), neem bark in equal quantities, 1 ounce to be taken for a dose, three times a day. Grape juice is also useful.

If there is Jaundice त्रिफला (Trifala), गुलबेल (Gulbel), दारु हलद (Daru halad), आणि कडु लिंब (Kadulimb) in equal parts; one ounce of this decoction to be taken three times a day.

According to Western science the average amount of blood in the body is 4.6 p.c. of the body weight. After loss of blood the vessels absorb liquid rapidly from the tissues and are soon filled again with blood the same in quantity but different in corpuscles and chemical constituents. In Pernicious Anaemea the quantity of blood is below the normal. The normal blood consists of plasma and blood corpuscles Red and White. Normal red corpuscles are large and small. White blood corpuscles in health present many varieties. Small and large lymphocytes are non-granular cells. Polymorpho nuclear leucocytes have granules. In some cells these granules stain with acid dyes in others with basic or neutral and in some cells with both acid and basic dyes.

Relative numbers in the blood are as follows:

Polymorpho-nuclear cells with neutrophyle granules 60-65 c.e.
-do-   with   large   eosionphile   granules   1-4   p.c.

Basophyle leucocytes ....0.3.1 p.c.
Small leucocytes..25 to 30 p.c.
Large lymphocytes ....3 to 6 p.c.

Marrow cells occur normally in red marrow of bone and in diseased conditions of blood. They look like large mononuclear leucocytes and have oval nucleus and possess four nucleoli. Blood platelets are round or oval bodies. They are faint yellow and granular and readily cling to blood corpuscles. All leucocytes have amoeboid movements.

Change in the disease: Red blood cells become fainter and irregular and show vacuoles or irregular points or knobs and their protoplasm take other stains besides eosin. White blood cells. Polomorpho-neucleus show greater division of neucleus with faint staining. In myelocytes the neucleus is swollen with vacuoles.

Deficiency in blood in general (corpuscles and haemoglobin) is called anaemia. Excess of blood in general is called plethora. In Anaemia—the skin is pale and waxy looking and also the mucus membrance.

The patient is weak and languid and have headaches, vertigo, fainting and ringing in the ears, murmurs. When this disease occurs among women between 14 and 24 it is called chlorosis. Blood corpuscles are below 60 p.c. and haemoglobin is only 25 p.c. In pernicious anaema; the skin acquires a yellow tint but the patient does not loose flesh; complains of dryness with loss of appetite. He gets fever. The blood is excessively pale and the red corpuscles are reduced but the haemoglobin is in excess. Colour index is greater than one.

Megalocytes are common and poikilocytes are numerous with neucleated red cells. White blood cells are less. In spleenic anaemia there is great enlargement of spleen with profound anaemia with enlargement of other lymphatic glands.

In Leucaemia— There is persistent increase in the number of white blood cells in the blood and the relations in the number of different leucocytes are greatly altered. In one variety Myelocytes are found in the blood to the extent of 30 or 40 p. c. and in other variety lymphocytes from 90 to 95 p. c.

Haemoglobin—Naemia—It arises when blood corpuscles are broken up in blood vessels so that haemoglobin escapes in the plasma giving it pink tinge. Urine is deep red.

Purpura—It is a diseased condition in which a number of haemorrhages occur in the skin so as to produce blotches of more or less purple colour.

Haemophylia—is a disease characterised by a tendency to excessive of uncontrollable bleeding either spontaneous or traumatic. It is cogenital and very often heriditary. Ayurveda does not distinguish the different forms of anaemia. All anaemia due to Vat are due to wasting diseases such as chronic fevers and other nerve disorders producing derangements in the digestive and assimilative processes in the body which tend to form less amount of blood. Anaemia is due to chronic constipation and other intestinal disorders fall under this head.

In all anemias due to derangement of Pitt there is fever more or less of distinct yellow tinge of the skin. Symptoms—more or less resemble the pernicious form.

Pitt disturbs the absorptive and assimilative processes which vitiate the blood and disintegrate. Red colouring matter if let loose in the skin giving rise to yellow tint. Patients complains of loss of appetite, and constipation, breathlessness and when Pitt is in excess it gives rise to fevers and profuse perspiration.

Anaemias due to derangement of Kuff; the patient is pale, skin smooth and moist and has generally good deal of cough and vomiting. He gets also occasionally diarrhoea with enlargement of external glands and of liver and spleen. The symptoms more or less resemble spleenic anemia.

In सन्निपात पांडुरोग–(Sannipat Pandurog): All the symptoms mentioned above are exaggerated. Urine is generally black or smoky with heamorrhages under the skin, diminution of vision, cough with abundant expectoration, palpitation, severe breathlessness, loss of appetite and severe diarrhoea. This arises owing to inco-ordination of Vat, Pitt and Kuff or to derangement of Vat and excessive formation of Pitt and Kuff. Symptoms more or less resemble. Haemoglobinaemia and Purpura.

Kidney 2/3 .... Diseases. From वाग्भट Vagbhta Diabetes insipidus and cerebral lesions in syphilis, emotional disturbances, injuries to the head etc. In these conditions urine is pale, sp. gr. 1002 to 1005.

इक्षु मेह (Ikshumeha): In this condition urine is like cane juice and sweet. It occurs in certain cases of dyspepsia arising from eating excess of sugar in the diet and want of exercise in fatty subjects; but in such cases the quantity is not increased.

सांद्र मेह (Sandra 3/2-Meha): In this case the urine is clear and quanity is normal; but gets thick after 24 hours. This is due to deposits of urates owing to cooling of the urine because they are soluble at body temperature and in concentrated urine due to inhealth, profuse perspiration and deficient intake of fluids, and in diseases such as heart affections which act by arterial low pressure in the renal circulation and in certain fevers, which lower arterial pressure and increase cutaneous and pulmonary transpiration of aqueous vapour and also in all conditions which increase the acidity of urine.

सुरा मेह (Sura Meha): In this condition the urine is liquid above and thick below. This generally occurs in the alkaline condition of urine from ingestion of much vegetable matter or food containing citrates, tratrates, nitrates of potassium and also afteer any large meal.

Urine also becomes alkaline from the presence of Ammonia due to bacterial decomposition of urea either within the bladder or to exposure to air in the vessel after standing.

पिष्ठ मेह (Pishta Meha): Urine is thick and white in this condition. This generally occurs in Cystitis with good deal of mucus and also in certain cases of tuberculous condition of kidney and bladder and also in disease called Phosphaturia. This occurs in alkaline condition of urine in the bladder.

शुक्र मेह (Shukra Meha): Here the urine contains whitish looking materials. These are either the secretions from the prostate or seminal glands. This is found in cases of general debility and diseases arising from excessive sexual intercourse. Here the seminal fluid becomes very thin and is secreted on the slightest stimulation such as the act of micturition and is mixed up with the urine.

सिकता मेह (Sikta Meha.): Here the urine contains sandy particles. This condition occurs in very acid urine due to precipitation of uric acid. Under the microscope they are distinguished by their yellow, orange or red colour.

Urates are precipitated in the amorphous form as a thick pink or red sediment. The urate deposits consists of urates of sodium, potassium and calcium. According to Ayurveda this मेह (Meha) is due to excess of पित्त (Pitt) in the body vitiating the blood flow.

शीत मेह (Sheet Meha): In this condition the urine is abundant and frequent and of sweetish smell. This generally occurs in diabetic urine. When ascetone, diascetic acid and oxybutyric acids are present, they also occur in certain acute fevers, gastro-intestinal affections, in advanced malignant disease, scurvy, eelampsia, psychical vomiting and delayed chloroform poisoning. According to Ayurveda this condition is due to excess of Kuff.

क्षार मेह (Kshar Meha): This is due to Ammoniacal decomposition of urine in bladder as occurs in retention of urine due to paralysis or atony of the organ in paraplegia and is certain nervous disorders.

नील मेंह (Neel Meha): This is due Inchean, the chromogen of Indigo-blue. It exists in normal urine to a very small extent, but is greatly increased in all conditions leading to retention of intentional contents. According to Ayurveda this is caused by derangement of Vat and Pitt causing intestinal disorders.

काल मेह (Kal Meha): In this condition the urine is black. This occurs in excessive haemolysis i.e. pernicious-anaemia, in diseases of liver. According to Ayurveda this is due to रक्त दोष (Raktdosh) i. e. derangement of blood and plasma.

रिंद्र मेह (Rindra Meha): Here the urine is deep yellow and the act of passing urine is painful. This occurs in mild form of cystitis and high fevers and in concentrated urine. This is due to (Pitt-dosh) पित्त दोष derangement of (Pitt) पित्त.

मंजिष्ट मेह (Mangist Meha): Here the urine contains blood and its derivatives. This occurs in Haemoglobinuria (Derangement of blood.) The urine is acid and deposits, on standing a dirty-brown sediment of epithelium, pigmented debries or corpuscles.

रक्त मेह (Rakta Meha) **Haematuria:** In this condition the urine contains blood, urine is light-red or dirty-brown. It occurs in stones and growths of the kidney.

मज्जा वसा (Majja and Vasa 3/2 Meha.) The urine contains fatty particles and chyle, as occurs in chyluris.

Here the urine is opaque, whitish or milky, on standing a layer of fat collects on the surface. This is due to obstruction of lymphatic vessels. Ayurveda attributes this to Rakt-Dosh derangement of blood and to excess of Kuff which obstructs the passge of (Rasas) रसाज body juices in to the circulatory system.

हस्ति मेह (Hasti Meha): In this condition the urine contains good deal of mucus as occurs in retention of urine from any cause. Ayuveda attributes this to derangement of (Wat) वात Saman Vayu which resides in stomach and intestines whose principal function is to regulate the process of assimilation and digestion of food and the separation of juices.

प्रमेह–**Prameh Disorders of Kidney, From** सुश्रुत

उदक मेह (Udak Meha): Urine is abundant, clear, and watery and without smell.

इक्षू मेह (Ikshu Meha): Urine is like cane juice and sweet.

सांद्र मेह (Sandra Meha): Urine gets thick after 24 hours.

सुरा मेह (Sura Meha): It is liquid above and thick at the bottom.

पिष्ट मेह (Pisht Meha): Urine is thick and white.

शुक्र मेह (Shukra Meha): Urine contains whitish looking material.

सिकता मेह (Sikta Meha): Urine contains sandy particles.

शीत मेह (Sheet Meha): There is frequencey of micturation and urine is abundant and sweetish smell.

शनै मेह (Shanai Meha): Urine is scanty and frequent.

क्षार मेह (Kshar Meha): Urine is alkaline and colour pale yellow.

नील मेह (Neel Meha): Urine is bluish.

काल मेह (Kal Meha): Urine is black.

रिंद्र मेह (Rindra Meha): It is yellow and micturition is painful.

मंजिष्ट मेह (Manjisht Meha): Urine is red, hot and foul.

रक्त मेह (Rakt Meha): It is red and micturition is painful.

मज्जार वसा मेह (Majjar Vasa Meha): Urine contains fatty particles.

हस्ति मेह (Hasit Meha): Micturition is very frequent and contains mucus.

मधु मेह (Madhu Meha): Urine is pale, watery looking and has a sweetish smell.

कफ मेह (Kuff Meha): Occurs from indigestion. There is vomiting, cough and cold.

पित्त मेह (Pitt Meha): There is fever, thirst, acid eructations, and diarrhoea.

वात मेह (Vat Meha): There is palpitation, colic, sleeplessness, breathlessness and cough.

प्रमेह (Prameha): Gives rise to various eruptions in the skin such as boils, carouncles.

Treatment—Little honey zi and हलद (Halad, grs 30 in one ounce of decoction of आंवला (Anwala) twice a day. One ounce of decoction of equal parts (one ounce of each in three pints of water) दारू हलद, देवदार (Daru halad, Devdar),

त्रिफला (Trifala) and नागरमोथा (Nagarmotha) or half a dramch of the juice of गुलबेल (Gul Bel) in little honey twice a day. सागर गोटा (Sagar Gota), रिंगणी (Ringni), कुड्या चे मुल (Kudia che Mul) खैरव बहावा (Khairav Bahawa) in equal parts to be powdered. 10 grains of the powder to be mixed in honey and taken twice a day. In मधु मेह (Madhu Meha) शिला जीत grs. x. (Shila jit) in little milk twice a day.

From वाग्भट Vagbhata.

Stones in the Kidneys and Bladder. अश्मरी (Ashmari): They generally occur in the children. They are of different varieties. Micturition is very painful and interrupted, and frequent. There is itching sensation round the anus and organs of generation. Urine is mixed with blood and the stream is bifurcated or narrowed. In बाताश्मरी (Watashmari the stone is black and its surface rough. In पित्ताश्मरी (Pittashmari) the stone is red or yellowish and in कफाश्मरी (Kafashmari) the stone is large, smooth and white. These give rise to symptoms of obstruction of urine and swelling over the region of the bladder. This is called मुत्रोदर (Mutrodar). When the bladder is more or less full due to obstruction of urine and when there is constant flow of urine it is called मुत्रोत्संग (Mutrotsang). When there is small tumour at the neck of the bladder it is called मूत्र-ग्रंथी (Mutra-granthi). When urine is mixed with semen and other secretions it is called मूत्र-शुक्र (Mutra-Shukra) and when it gives bad smell it is called विड्वीधात (Vidvighat). When it occasions good deal of pain after exercise and when micturition is frequent and when it is reddish looking the disorder is called उष्णावात (Ushanavat) and when the urine is whitish in colour the disorder is called मूत्रसाद (Mutrasad.)

AFFECTIONS OF THIE BLADDER

वातिक मूत्र कृच्छः (Watik mutra Krchh)—There is pain in the abdomen, rectum and scrotum, scanty and repeated micturition.

पितिक (Pittik) form—There is painful micturition and urine is red and reddish-yellow and in कफजन्य मूत्र कृच्छ (Kuff janya krchh) there is inflammation of bladder and rectum, frequency of micturition and urine is scanty and mucoid, and in त्रिदोशात्मक मूत्र कृच्छ (Tridoshatmak mutra krchh)—All these symptoms are exaggerated and when urine gets more or less concentrated in bladder through Vat, Pitt and Kuff it produces different kinds of stones mentioned above. *Treatment:* 3/4 Fomentation over the affected part, decoction of barley and कुलीथ (Kulith) and light diet are useful in allaying the pain.

ज्येष्ट मध आनि दारू हळद (Jaisthmadh and Daru halad). In equal parts, decoction of this to be mixed with rice water and one ounce of this should be taken twice a day to relieve the pain. When there are symptoms of stone forming aperient diuretic and disphoretic medicines are useful. Seeds of करंज, अंकोल, निवली, साग व कमल (Karanj, Ankol, Nivlee, Sag or Kamal) one grain each to be powdered and mixed in sugar and taken in hot water. This dissolves small stones and facilitates expulsion through urine and so also the decoction of one ounce of the root of शेवगा (Shevga).

Til, अघाड़ा, केळ, पळस आनि जव (Aghara, Ker, Palas and Jav) 10 grs each to be burnt and the ashes mixed in goats milk and should be taken twice a day. This medicine is useful in dissolving small stones. If this does not dissolve the small stones, operative treatment becomes necessary.

According to Western science the average quantity of urine per day is 50 ounces, sp. gr. is between 1015 to 1025 and solids amount to about 950 grains, out of the total solids half the amount is urea. It forms normally about 2 p. c. of urine and besides it contains chlorides, sulphates, phosphates. The daily excretion of uric acid is from 8 to 15 grains and other solids. Pale urine is of low sp. gr. and contains large quantity of water and less amount of solids. High coloured urines are scanty, of great density and contain more solids. Reaction of urine is faintly acid. Diseases of urine are classed as follows.

The inflammation of kidney, acute, chronic or interstitial. Red granular kidney and lardacious kidney. They produce albuminurea, blood in the urine, casts dropsy, changes in the heart, changes in the eyes, secondary inflammations and uraemia. In acute form the dropsy is sudden, urine scanty and thick with albumin and turbid, with casts. It is generally red in colour. In the chronic form urine is scanty, general dropsy with effusions into the serous cavities, chronic interstetial nephritis occurs in two forms. Pale granular kidney there is no dropsy with plenty of albumia and amount of urine is normal. The patient suffers from headache and pulse is of high tension. Red granular-kidney onset very slow. There is abundant pale urine and of low sp. gr. Albumin is very small in quantity. It is quite clear. There is slight oedema of the eye-lids. The heart and pulse reveal changes in the circulation. Suppurative nephritis there is chill with fever and the urine contains pus, mucus, blood or albumin. The urine is often abundant with no diminution of urea. Lardacious disease of the kidney such as occurs in tuberculosis or syphilis. The urine is in excess in the beginning and afterwards it becomes scanty—There is dropsy. In Tubercular kidney urine is acid with abundant deposit of pus and contains blood from time to time and sometimes the urine is ammoniacal and ropy. In Renal calculus—The urine is acid and scanty and frequent and accompanied with good deal of pain at the time of passing water.

In Bacillurin—The urine is often clear when passed, but on standing it deposits a layer like mucus at the bottom, above this there is a haze or turbidity and at the top clean layer. Urine is always acid and it does not become clear either with heat, ascetic acid or alkalies and has a peculiar offensive odour which is not ammoniacal—Under microscope pus cells and numerous bacilli are found.

Tumours of kidneys such as sarcoma, carcinoma etc. may also disturb the quantity of urine. It may contain blood, albumin and pus but in some cases it may remain perfectly normal in quality, density, and colour, but frequently it contains blood and cancer cells. Sometimes there is albumin also.

Ayurveda describes various kinds of प्रमेह (Prameha). These are all due to derangements of Vat, Pitt and Kuff. Derangements from Vat are purely nervous, for example polyuria in Hysteria goes under the name of उदकमेह (Udakmha) where urine is abundant, clear and watery. This abundance of urine also occurs in certain brain conditions such as in some cases of cerebral tumours, fright.

शोफ (Shoph) *Inflammation.*

Deranged Vayu, Pitt and Kuff flow through blood and irritate the skin and organs and cause disorder in the normal flow of blood and thus causing stasis and consequent inflammation. Various digestive troubles arising from eating acid, sour, saltish and pungent foods, bad quality of meat, indigestion, diarrhoea, piles and fevers cause irritation of various दोश (Dosha) in the chest, abdomen, and bladder, produce inflammation in different parts. The inflammation caused by irritated Vayu causes boils and dryness of the skin and when due to Pitt it is reddish, painful and hot and produces fever and when due to Kuff the part is not hot and does not itch. The inflammation is hard and thick when pressed it produces itch and takes some time to heal and very little blood flows on incision. In त्रिदोश (Tridosha) inflammation has all the symptoms mentioned above. The inflammation due to wounds, ulcers and irritants is called अभिघातक (Abhighatak) it is hot, red, painful. Poisonous inflammation due to bites from various animals comes very quickly and it is very hot and painful.

विसर्प (Visarp): Arises from inflammation from wounds and it is divided according to predominence of symptoms of Vat, Pitt and Kuff and when due to all three they produce very servere symptoms such as fever, delirium, pains in the limbs and joints and cause destruction of the surrounding parts and gangrene, ulcers of various kinds also cause विसर्प (Visarp) called क्षत विसर्प (Kshat Visarp).

Treatment—Fasting or light diet and mild purgative.

Local treatment—Lime-seed, meal poultice and fomentation.

In Vat Shoph—Castor oil as purgative is beneficial.

Nimb tree bark, पुनर्नवा, करंज (Punarnava, Karanj)—and Madar leaves in equal parts, one ounce each to be well pounded and applied over the affected part or निली तुलस, हलद, कलौंजी जिरे (Nily, Tulas, Halad, Kalauji jeere) in equal parts acts also well.

Infusion made of सुंठ (Sunth) ginger two dramchs, Chiretta one ounce in three pints of water, one ounce to be taken twice a day. Baths of water containing neem, पुनर्नवा, करंज (Punarnava, Karanj) and madar leaves are good in reducing inflammation of the skin. An infusion made out of ज्येष्ट मध, कटुकी, हिरडे, दारूहलद पिंपली (Jaist Madh, Katuki, Hirde, Daruhalad Pipely) one ounce of each in 6 pints of water, one ounce should be takan twice a day.

गुल बेल	(Gul bel)	One ounce	To be powdered
हिरडे	(Hirde)	One ounce	10 grains of these
पुनर्नवा	(Punarna)	Four drachms	to be taken twice
गुग्गु	(Gugul)	One drachm	a day. They act as alternative.

Treatment of विसर्प (Visarp): Fasting, and mild purgatives should be given in the beginning. An emetic made out of decoction ज्येष्टमध (Jaist madh) इंद्र जव (Indra jav) and आणि गेलफल (Gelful) in equal proportion in six pints of water one ounce of each may be taken and one ounce of this decoction given as an emetic early in the morning or decoction made out of grapes and त्रिफला (Trifala) one ounce may be given.. External application of well pounded young sprouts of Banian tree, plantain tree, and seed of lotus in water and mixed with *ghee*. It acts well in विसर्प (Visarp) due to Pitt and in Kuff Visarp. External application of त्रिफला (Trifala), पद्मकाष्ट (Padmakasht), वाला (Bala) and आणि कण्हेर (Kanher) well powdered in water and mixed in गेरू (Geru) also reduces the inflammation. When the glands are enlarged an external application of bark of शेवगा (Shewga), करंज (Karanj), Radish and बेहडे (Behade) pounded in hot water is useful or making nut juice 10 drops, हिराकस (Hirakas) ferri-sulph zii दालचिनी (Dalchini) cinnamon zi, to be well pounded and lastly venesection.

According to Western science the inflammation is a process of degeneration and regeneration. If the process continues it tends to lead to suppuration in a cavity it turns into abscess and if on the surface it becomes an ulcer. Inflammation when it causes death of the tissue it becomes gangrene. It occurs anywhere in the body. The inflammed part is red hot, swollen and painful and its function is deranged. These five signs are seen more or less in inflammation of mucus, membrane, serous membranes and deep seated organs.

Predisposing Causes: Impairment of quality of blood by deviation from normal metabolism, by insufficient or improper food or air or by morbid state such as anaemia, diabetes, and gout, tuberculosis etc. or from poisoning by lead, mercury etc. or by impediment in circulation, such as weak heart or by arterial or venous obstruction. Disease or injury of a nerve trunk disturbing the trophic function. The prominent symptom of any severe inflammation are fever with diminished secretion in the glandular organs, causing scanty urine, dryness of mouth etc. Increased pulse rate and nerve disturbances such as headache delirium etc. when the inflammation subsides there is cessation of the activity of the cause and its removal from the body and normal circulation of blood through the affected part.

Ayurveda attributes fever to the excess of (Pitt) पित्त in the blood causing derangement of the circulation in the part and this excess of Pitt or its derangement in the production of various glands of the parts. Redness, swelling and pain and derangement of the function of the part is considered to be due to वात दोष (Vat dosh). Derangement of Vat i.e. derangement of the nerves supplying these parts.

Ayurveda also believes that these inflammation may occur anywhere in the body causing inflammations of the organs such as tungs: causing नव ज्वर ((navajwar) (nine days fever called Pneumonia), liver (hepatites), kidneys etc. These also may form suppuration and ulcers in the system suppuration destroys the tissue of the organ and forming ulcers as occurs in Tubercular processes in various organs and malignant ulcers of the skin, tongue etc.

Chapter IX

From वाग्भट Vagbhata

कुष्ट (Kushta) and आणि क्रुमी (Krumi) Skin diseases and diseases caused by worms.

दोषा (Doshas): Arising from digestive troubles and bad quality of food vitiate and increase the quantity of Pitt in the system. This Pitt vitiates the blood and Vat which in turn irritates the skin, muscles etc. and cause various kinds of inflammations on the skin. These कुष्ट (Kushtas) are of seven kinds. Before skin diseases begin there is generally dryness or roughness of the skin, profuse perspiration, or no perspiration, discolouration, itching and redness.

कापाल कुष्ट (Kapal Kushta) is blackish or reddish looking, rough and edges superficial and irregular.

औंदुबर कुष्ट (Audumber Kushta) is red with raised edges and in which blood and pus is thick and it is hot and painful.

मंडल कुष्ट (Mandal Kushta): It is hard, white or red in colour raised and round itching edges, yellowish with profuse flow.

विचर्चिका (Vicharchika): It is full of lymph and inflammed and itching.

ऋक्ष जिव्ह (Riksh Jivha): It is rough and raised with red edges and blackish in the centre which is very painful and covered with small boils.

चर्म कुष्ट (CharmaKushta): It is rough like the skin of an elephant.

किटिभ (Kitibh): It is rough, very itching and black.

सिध्मकुष्ट (SidhmaKushta): Tinia versicolour—It is yellowish brown in colour whitish scales are easily detached by scraping patches extend and fresh ones are formed.

It generally occurs on the covered parts, neck, chest and abdomen.

विपादिका (Vipadika): Occurs on the hands and feet and cause deep fissures which are painful and itchy and covered with red papules.

दद्रु (Dadroo) Ring-worm: It is superficial, itching, slightly raised.

शतारू (Shataru): Generally occurs on the joints. It is very painful and red surrounding parts inflamed.

पुंडलीक (Pundalik): It is red at the edges and white in the centre, hot and painful, full of lymph and blood.

विस्पोट (Vispot): Small red irregularly spread boils.

पामा (Pama): Small reddish looking eruptions in hands elbow, buttocks, painful and full of itch.

चर्मदल (Charmadal) : They are painful boils which are hot and itchy.

कांकन कुष्ट (Kankan Kushta): It is very hot and painful. It is red as गुंज (Gunj) and inflamed.

स्पर्शे काहार शय्यादि सेवनात्रा- यशोगदाः ।
सर्वे संचारिणो नेत्रत्वग्विकारा विशेषतः ।।

वाग्भट निदान अध्याय 14 श्लोक 41: ।

Touch, eating in the same dish or sleeping in the same bed spread the diseases. Out of these, eye diseases and skin diseases are very contagious.

Treatment—At first mild aperients and emetics should be given.

वावडींग (Wavding)	four tolas.
आवलकठी (Auvalkathi)	"
हिरडे (Hirde)	"
निशोत्तर (Nishottar)	12 tolas
गुळ (Guda)	48 tolas

Make three grain pill and one pill twice a day for a month. Decoction of the following:

हळद (Halad)	one ounce
खैर (Khair)	"
नीम बरक (Neem bark)	"
देवदार (Devdar)	"
Water	4 pints

One ounce to be taken twice a day.

External application of बांळत लिंब, हळद, दारूहळद, तुळस, शेवका, शिरस, धने, चंदन आनि किरमनी ओवा. (Balant limb, Halad, Daruhalad, Tulas, Sevka, Shiras, Dhane, Chandan and Kirmany owa) in equal parts to be well pounded and applied to the skin. मेन (Men) Wax ZI. शेंदुर (Shendur) ZI. गुगुल (Guggul) ZI, Copper sulph grs. X. शीरस (Shiras) oil ZI.

This ointment is very useful.

कोड़ (Kod) *Leucoderma and treatment.*

Marking nuts four—

निवडुंग (Nivdung) cactus four drachms, to be well pounded and applied over the affected part or बावची (Bowchi) seeds 16 tolas, हरताळ (Hartal) four tolas, to be well rubbed in four ounces of fat or butter and applid over the affected part. Hide of elephant or panther should be burnt and ashes mixed in oil and applied.

Bark of black उबंर (Umber) tree 2 ozs. and बेहड़ा (Behda) 2 oz. should be boild and mixed with Bowchi seeds one tola and applied.

According to Western science the skin is liable to the same diseases as other organs, Cutaneous haemorrhages called echymosis. Papules are red or pink elevations of the skin. Vesicles are small blisters and bullae large vehicle and they become pustules when they contain pus. A circumcised oedema of the skin is called wheal, and when there is loss of substance it is called ulcer. Skin diseases are inflammatory in origin due to toxins circulating in the blood and others are due to micro-organisms acting locally. They go under the name of Erythema, Urticaria, Pemphygus and Herpes.

Eczema—is a superficial inflammation of the skin producing visication and followed by destruction of the superficial part and secretion of serum, and when the skin presents bran like appearance it is called Pityreasis. Red white patches covered with scales is Psoriasis. When the eruption is papular it is called lichen and if accompanied with severe itching it is Prurigo. Diseases of the skin due to micro-organisms, Impetigo. This is infection of eczema with pyogenic organisms.

Tuberculosis of skin Lupus.

New growths on the skin such as fibroma molluscum cheloid xanthoma.

Hypertrohies of the skin are produced by friction and pressure. They are callosity and corn. In Ichthyosis, the skin is dry and rough and warts are small exeresceuces from the skin. The skin in seleroderma is hard tense and atrophic. Besides skin also undergoes alterations of pigment such as leucoderma.

Sweat glands in the skin also undergo changes. Anidrosis that is deficiency of perspiration. Hyperidrosis that is excess of perspiration. Diseases of sebacious glands cause seborrhoea that is excessive secretion of sebum and Acne is caused by the blocking of their secretion. Boils and carbuncles are caused by local infection of staphylococus. Pyogenes diseases of the hair cause alopacia. Besides skin is also invaded by vegetable parasites giving rise to Tinia versicolour ringworm, favns. Animal parasites cause scabies, pediculosis.

Ayurveda attributes the origin of all skin diseases to excess of Pitt circulating in the blood which irritates the skin. It tends to retard the capillary circulation by diminishing the activity, of the cells contained in the skin thus producing circumcised inflammations. By derangement of Pitt in stomach and intestines it produces digestive disorders which vitiate the blood giving rise to skin eruptions.

Pitt also exists in Ras Dhatu which is formed by mixture of food juices and blood. When its proportion is in excess of the requirement it produces irritation and itching sensation of the skin. It also exists in small quantity in heart muscle when this is out of proportion it deranges the circulation in the skin producing disorders. It also exists to some extent in the skin, where it helps to regulate the heat of the body.

Any derangement here causes excessive or diminished perspiration. Large and small boils are caused by excessive formation of Pitt in the skin causing localized inflammation and when a boil is large and has a tendency to spread causing destruction of tissue underneath it becomes a carbuncle.

Chapter X

Worms and Germs कृमी (Krimi)

There are four kinds. (1) Those that arise from (mal) मल (2) those from Kuff, (3) from blood, and (4) from vegetables. Worms that are produced from matters outside are lice and bugs and produce papules, small blebs and itch on the skin.

Worms arising from (Kuff janya) कफजन्य are produced from eating sweets, milk, curd and new rice and पुरीश जन्य (Purish jania) from eating raw vegetables.

कफजन्य (Kuff jania) worms reside in the intestinal tract they are either white or red and are of seven kinds. अंत्राद (Antrad), उदर विष्ट (Uder wisht), हृदयाद (Rhudyad), महाकुह (Mahakuh), कुरू (Kuru), दर्भकुसुम (Durbhkhusum) and सुगन्ध (Sugandh) and cause salivation, vomiting, tastelessness, fever, distension of abdomen, sneezing and cold and digestive troubles.

रक्त जन्य कृमी (Rakt janya krimi) reside in vessels conveying blood. They are very minute without feet, round and red. Some of them are very minute and invisible. They are of six kinds केशाद (Keshad) लोभ विध्वन्स (Lobh widhwans), लोभ द्वीप (Lobh dweep), उडंबर (Udambar), सौरस (Sowras) आणि and मातृक (Matrik), पुरीष जन्य (Purush janya) कृमी (Krimi) they are in the small and large intestines. They travel downwards and cause eruptions and breathlessness and colic and foul breath, some are flat and round, some are thin and slender and they are either yellow, white or reddish in colour.

They cause diarrhoea, colic, distension of abdomen, thinness, roughness and paleness of the skin and itching sensation round the anus.

Treatment—Fast for a day or two or very light food, mild emetic and aperient, afterwards enema of decoction of बावडींग (Bawding). In worms due to external मल (Mul) such as lice etc. good bath and an aperient to be given and ointment of Gandhak (sulphur) and decoction of Palus पलस seeds.

(पलास) Palas seeds well pounded 2 drachms.

Water ... ... 2 pints.

One ounce of decoction to be taken twice a day or बावडींग (Bawding) 4 drachms पिंपली (Pipeli) 4 drachms मिरे (Mire) 4 drachms त्रिफला (Trifala) 4 drachms water ... 3 pints.

One ounce of this to be taken twice a day.

According to Western science the worms found in the intestines are round worms. It is about 10 inches long, female is little longer. They are found in the faeces of the host. They cause nausea, foul breath, irregular appetite, abdominal pain and itching at the nose. They are pink cylindrical and tapering at each end. They inhabit the small intestines. *Tapeworm.* It also inhabits the small intestines. They are recognized by the discovery of small segments in the faeces. They cause colic, irregular appetite, and deficient or voracious appetite, salivation and itching at the nose.

Whip worm: This produces anaemia, the result of taxius causing haemolysis and acting upon the bone marrow.

Thread-worms: They cause local symptoms at the anus that is heat and itching at the anus worse at night also irritability of bladder and frequent micturition in children.

Hook-worm: They are small worms. The female is 1/2 inch in length and the male 1/3rd. They attach themselves to the mucus-membrane of the upper part of Intestines. They produce very severe anaemia and also occasional skin eruptions of papule or wheals.

Ayurveda describes these worms to be of seven kinds and they arise from eating raw vegetables and sweets.

Besides these Ayurveda describes several bacteria that reside in blood. They are either round or red, very minute and invisible. According to Western science several parasites also reside in blood and cause diseases such as malarial parasities. These are protoplasmic bodies seen in red blood corpuscles. They enlarge and occupy more and more of red cell granules of pigment accumulate in their interior, then the pigment aggregates in the centre of the organisms which then loses its amaeboid character. The process of segmentation takes place first at the nucleus and at the same time both these and pigment granules are set free in the blood plasma.

The specific micro-organism of Typhoid is a bacillus 2-3 Micron in length with round ends and provided from 8 to 12 fine flagella twice its length. It is found in the blood, sputum, urine and faeces. In the Mediterranean fever specific organism is a micro-coccus which can be obtained from the blood, urine and faeces.

Influenza bacillus is a minute rod 1-5 Micron, found in sputum and blood of patients suffering from it.

Bacillus of plague is a short rod with rounded ends flagellated and stains more deeply at the ends and is generally found in the blood, in the inflammed glands, faeces, urine and sputum.

Staphylococcus and strepto-coccus organisms are found in the blood in septaecemia and Pyaemia. Diplococcus

Pneumonia of Frankel is found in blood in severe cases. Lower bacteria are all minute cellular bodies devoid of nucleus and they take stains. They occur in several forms minute, spherical and ovoid bodies are called coccii or micro-coccii, straight rod like bodies are bacilli. Spiral forms are called spirella coccii in threads are strepto-coccii, in plates merismopedia is cubes sarcina and when grouped in irregular manner staphylo-coccii and when coccii or rods are united with gelatinous matter, they are called zooglea. Some bacilli possess clia for movement.

Micro-organisms: These micro-organisms are reproduced by division or by the formation of spores.

Higher bacteria belonging to the class of Trichomycetae cause also infectious diseases. They are of greater size and consist of filaments of simple cells and have special organs of reproduction in the cells called Gonidia. They are Thiothrix Leptothrix Cladothrix and Streptothrix.

Few infectious diseases are caused by organisms belonging to animal kingdom. They are entamoeba of dysentery haemoeba of malaria, trypanosoma of sleeping sickness. Some pathogenic bacteria thrive on the living and animal tissues, some flourish in dead and dying animal tissue and in vegetable and inorganic matter. They are called saprophytes. In some diseases only one pathogenic micro-organism is found such as anthrax and syphilis and in others more than one are detected as in pneumonia, septecaemia etc.

Diseases produced by micro-coccii are Septecaemia Pyaemia, Erysipelas, Cerebro spinal fever, Pneumonia etc.

From Bacillii-Enteric cholera, plague, Tubercle etc. From Fungi-Actino-mycosis, myectoma and diseases of the skin etc.

From Protozoa-Malarial fevers, amoebic dysentery, Kalaazar, Relapsing fever.

The following diseases of the skin are due to vegetable parasites. Tenia versicolour, Fungi consist of jointed rods or threads the mycelial and round of oval bodies spores. They are connected with the hairs.

Ring-worm—The fungus is called Trichophyton microsporon. The shaft of the hair is penetrated by the mycelial threads. The other fungus is called Trichophyton megatosporun. Animal parasites of the skin.

Acarus scabies is oval in shape 1/70 inch long and provided with suckers or stalks and behind with long bristles. The pediculi cause itching and pustular eczema. The head louce is 2 millimeter long and one millimeter broad and breeds among the hair of scalp. Body louce is slightly bigger. They cause pruritus. The crab louce is smaller than the above two. They cause eczematous eruption.

Now Ayurveda states that some parasites are external in origin and reside in connection with hair and clothes and give rise to itching, boils, local inflammations. They are small and have feet. They are described as follows in वाग्भट (Vaghbhata).

तिल प्रमाण संस्था न वर्णाः । केशांबरा श्रयाः । ।
बहु पादाश्च सुक्ष्माश्च । युका लिक्षाश्च नामतः । ।
वाग्भट निदान स्थान अध्याय १४ श्लोक १/४१
Waghbut Nidana sthan Chapter 14 verse 44
उवा आणि लिखा निदान स्थान अध्याय १४ श्लोक ४४
स्पर्सें काहार शय्यादि । सेवनात् प्राय शोगदाः । ।
सर्वे संचारिणो नेत्रत्व । ग्विकारा विशेषतः ।
वाग्भट निदान स्थान अध्याय १४ श्लोक ४४
Vagbhata Nidana sthan Chapter 14 verse 41

Translation: Touch, eating in one dish and sleeping in one bed communicate diseases from one to another and among them Eye and Skin diseases are specially contagious.

कफ जन्य कृमी (Kuff janya krimi) that is the worms that arise from (Kuff) कफ. Ayurveda says that these arise from taking improper and unsuitable food and from eating sweet foods, bad quality of milk and new rice of bad quality. These generally reside in the intestines. Some of them are flat, some are hooked and small and look like sprout of a germinating seed and they are either long or short and white or red in colour and they cause salivation, indigestion, tastelessness, fainting, vomiting, distention of stomach, colic, thinness, sneezing and cold.

They are probably tapeworms and those that cause thinness and anaemia are hook worms.

कफादामाये शये जाता वृद्धाः । सर्पन्ति सर्वतः ।
पृथुव घ्रनिभा । केचित केचिदंडू पदोयमाः । ।
निदान स्थान वाग्भट अध्याये १४ श्लोक १४

Vagbhata Nidana sthan Chapter 14 verse 47.

पुरीष जन्य कृमी (Purish janya Krumi worms.)

These are vegetable parasites and give rise to Ringworm, Teniaversicolour etc. Acteno-mycosis, Myectoma etc.

They also reside in the intestinal tract and they travel downwards towards the rectum and give rise to foul breath and eructations. They are either flat or round, flat slender or thick and are yellow, white or black in colour. They cause diarrhoea, colic, thinness, dryness of skin, anaemia and itching sensation at the anus. They are thread worms.

रक्त जन्य (Rakta janya) germs are those that reside in the blood. They are small without feet, round and red and some of them are so minute that they are invisible and they produce different kinds of diseases. They are different kinds of pathogenic micro-organisms mentioned in Western science producing fevers.

रक्त वाहि शिरोत्याना । रक्त जा जंत वोडणवः ।
अपादा वृत्त ताम्राश्च । सौभ्श्यात्के चिद दर्शनाः ।।
केशादा लोभ विध्वन्सा । लोभ द्वीपा उदुबराः ।
षट्ते कुष्टैक कर्माण । सह सौर समातरः ।।
(निदान स्थान वाग्भट अध्याय १४)

They are of six kinds called (Keshad) केशाद Lomevidhwance (लोभ विध्वंस), Lomedwip (लोभ द्वीप), Udumber (उदंबर), Souras (सौरस) and Matrk (मातृक).

Disprdes of Vat (वात) Disorders of Central-Nervous-system. They are generally nervous disorders such as neuralgia, paralysis, sciatica, headaches, hemiplegia, paraplegia and cerebral-haemorrhage etc.

When Vayu is in excess in the stomach and intestinal tract, it causes disorders of digestion such as diarrhoea, distension etc. It should be treated with emetics and mild purgatives or enema when in the head causing headaches and neuralgia massage and various kinds of oils mixed with camphor are useful when the skin is affected, hot baths and fomentations and when acting on blood tonics and good digestible food.

If there be loss of sensation over any part, massage with rock salt and oil after fomentation.

The infusion of कुलीथ (Kulith), जव (Jav) आणि and बहावा (Bahawa) an ounce of each in three pints of water, one ounce to be taken twice a day or त्रिफळा (Trifala), चवक (Chavak), कटुकी (Katuki), पिंपली (Pipeli), नागर मोथा

(Nagarmotha) to be well pounded 2 dramch eath. 10 grains of each in one tea spoon full of honey twice a day.

Treatment: वात रक्त (Vat Rukt)—Slight venesection is very beneficial. Old ghee one drachm, infusion of grapes and mahuwa flower one ounce three times a day, and when there are pains all over the body enema is good.

When (Vat Rakt) वात रक्त is due to Kuff.

Grapes dried	... ...	one ounce.
हलद (Hald)	... ...	one drachm.
त्रिफला (Trifala)	... ...	one drachm.
Water	... ...	3 Pints.

One ounce of this in little honey twice a day is useful. External application of Til (तिल) and milk. When due to derangement of Kuff fomentation and external application of बेखंड (Bekhand), कोष्ट (Kosht), बड़ी साप (Badisap), हलद (Halad), आणि and दारू (Daru) हलद (Halad).

Relieves the pain or seed of (Sheewga) शेवगा well pounded and boiled in rice कंजी (Kanji).

Diet should be light and nutritious, according to Western science diseases of the nervous system are the disorders of brain spinal cord and nerves which manifest themselves through the functions of motion, sensation special sense intellect and emotions. Ayurveda says that (Vat) वात gives all power to the body mechanism. It has the power of taking food into the mouth to the stomach intestines. It aids in the digestion and separation of the juices from the excreta. It also aids to carry the juices of the body to the different tissues. In fact it practically performs the functions of central nervous system mentioned in the Western science. Western science says that nerve tissue is a kind of protoplasm with highly specialized properties i.e. excitability acting under a stimulus. Depression is the effect of less energy than ordinary.

Nervous system is built up of nerve centres with an excitable surface on one side and with organs of force on the other. Impression disturbs this excitable surface and excites it to action by a molecular change in the associated nerve endings. This impulse is conducted by efferent nerve through posterior root ganglion to the spinal cord, from which it is again reflected out through efferent nerves and tracts as an impulse to the organs of force-muscles, glands, vessels etc. This process is called reflex action. Nerve protoplasm is also automatic. The highest centres are the seat of emotions, intellect, will and consciousness. They reside in the convolutions in the cortex of the brain. Similar automatic and reflex centres are in the basal ganglia, cerebellum, medulla and cord and the whole constitutes a series of successive centres joined to each other by tracts which conduct, associate and co-ordinate the impulses. The peripheral ganglia, the sympathetic are chiefly automatic in its action. Viscera such as heart, lung, liver, kidney etc. and vessels are governed by centres in the medulla and cord, the mechanism of which is partly reflex. They are also constantly influenced by impressions from outside. Efferent nerves between the centres and viscera are derived from the medulla and partly from the sympathetic chain. Besides this the viscera have intrinsic local ganglia automatic in action but partially controlled by higher centres. Sensation is a cerebral state. It originates in the periphery. Impression is, therefore, a sensation which may or may not travel onwards into a still higher part of the cerebrum (brain) where it becomes a perception, which is a part of consciousness.

The tissues and organs in health are sensitive but they do not originate sensations. A slight disturbance is sufficient to arouse perception of the condition of the organ. There is, therefore, constant existence of general sensibility.

Motion: It is an act of muscular contraction caused by stimulation of any part of efferent or motor side from the cortex of the brain to the muscle itself. Contraction is also effected by stimulation of some part of sensory side reflected through lower centres in the cord. Ayurveda does not define thoroughly the functions of (Vat) वात but it is considered as one of the principals generating power in the body required to maintain the body in the proper state of body mechanism. Ayurveda considers this principal factor of life as something which is invisible. It is an atomic force. Atoms are now further divided into something which are constantly in motion. Animal body also consists of atoms. This movement of atoms change, irritation and disinterration is constantly going on. The factor that is continuously causing this electrical and vibratory motion of the invisible parts of atoms is Vayu. The protoplasm of the central nervous system is very sensitive to this motion and is acted on first. In visible motion of the invisible components of atoms composing the nerve protoplasm is started in the substance which gathers strength and acceleration as it travels through different tracts, ganglia centres and nerves until it becomes sufficiently strong as to cause visible changes in the organs to which it reaches. The protoplasm of the cells of the different structures of which the body is composed are not so delicate as the nerve cells and require stronger force to set their action in motion. This (Vat) वात is generated in the body by the action of the invisible parts of the atoms themselves and acted on by external influences and as well as from the actions and reactions of the food substances that are daily taken in the body. When this (Vat) वात is deranged, vitiated or aggravated in one particular part of the body it stimulates or errilates the nerve protoplasm of the nerves supplying these parts and produces paralysis pain, inflammation or other circulatory changes in the part supplied by the nerves. Ayurveda further says that this Vat (force) resides specially in certain parts of the body.

First is प्राण वायु (Pran uayu) principally resides in head, neck and chest i.e. performs motor, sensory, circulatory, respiratory and other functions of that part. All diseases of the brain such as cerebral haemorrhage, encephalitis meningitis and tumours. General paralysis of the insane, cholera, epilepsy, migrane, vertigo, paralysis, agitans, tetanus. Hysteria etc. arise from its disorders: It also affects the circulation, respiration, salvation, mastication and other disorders affecting the centres situated in that region. Diseases of the medulla such as bulber paralysis, compressions and tumours.

Western science has described minutely localization of functions and effects of lesions in the brain. Ayurveda does not speak about these but all the diseases arising from them are classed as one and attributed to disorders of Vat (वात) in that region.

Western science divides the brain into motor and sensory areas. Irritative lesions cause convulsions and destructive paralysis. Motor area is defined round the fissure of Rolando in which centres for the face, arm and legs are found.

Fibres from these pass to the base of brain through internal capsule and decussate in the medulla. Sensory tract passes through the posterior part of the internal capsule from the spinal cord and medulla and reaches the sensory centres in the post central convolutions. Ayurveda does not describe these tracts nor its functions.

According to Ayurveda उदानवायु (Udan vayu). regulates the functions of the chest, nose, neck, speech, expiration and remembrance. All nerve diseases arising in these parts are attributed to its disorder. Asthma, whooping-cough, palpitation of the heart and its other functional disorders—disorders of speech, act of respiration, dysphonia;

disorders of the functions of the muscles in those region as mentioned in Western science are attributed to its disorder. It corresponds to the respiratory centre in the medulla as mentioned in Western science.

व्यानवायु (Vyan vayu) regulates the functions of the heart and motor functions of the muscles of the rest of the body. It corresponds to the cardiac centre in the medulla as mentioned in the Western science.

समानवायु (Saman wayu): It is the nerve mechanism which is concerned in the assimilation and disgestion of the food. Nervine disorders such as constipation arising from less peristalic action of the intestines paralysis, are attributed to this. Its centre is situated in the middle of the spinal cord.

अपानवायु (Apan vayu): It deals with the mechanism of micturition, defaecation and sexual organs. Its centre is in the lower region of spinal cord and its disorder produces either irritative or paralytic symptoms of bladder, rectum and sexual organs.

Western science says that paralysis that is loss of power in the muscles is due to lesion in the nervous system. Ayurveda attributes these to the disordered action of vayu which stops all impulses going to the muscles which cause its contractions. *Spasms*—are morbid involuntary muscular contractions. They are either interrupted or continuous. All clonic convulsions such as seen in epilepsy, uraemia, puerperal-eclampsia, organic cerebral disease are attributed by Ayurveda to the irritation caused by (Vayu) वायु in the system. In spasmodic wry neck and in spasmodic tics these spasms consist of sharp contractions of more isolated muscles with slower relaxations. Athetosis slow movements of small muscles at the distal extremities of limbs.

Tremors are tremblings in which ossilations of the part occur with alternate contraction and relaxation of the antogonistic muscles. They are seen in nervous emotions, muscular exhaution, paralysis agitans, mercurial and lead poisoning.

Ayurveda attributes these to the deviation of the force (Vat) वात, (Udan vayu) उदान वायु causing slight irritation and inco-ordination of muscles used in particular movements. These movements are checked to some extent by the effort of the will as occurs in disseminated sclerosis, when force generated by (Pran vayu) प्राण वायु is in excess.

Tonic convulsions as seen in Tetanus, Hysteria, meningitis etc. are due to (Vat) वात according to Ayurveda when it irritates the whole nervous system.

Vayu also generates energy in the muscles which cause their contraction, by causing continuous catabolic changes. Thus all diseases of muscles which cause increase or diminution of energy are attributed to the disordered function of (Vayu) वायु as seen in Progressive-muscular atrophy. According to Ayurveda Vayu also regulates the nerves of the skin which assists in keeping the body temperature constant.

According to Western science this mechanism consists of governing centre in the brain called heat regulating centre which is the function of (Pran vayu) प्राण वायु.

Efferent sensory nerves carry from the skin the impressions of heat and cold to the (Pran vayu) प्राण वायु which is the chief centre, which regulates the (Vyan-vayu) व्यानवायु the centre which regulates the function of the heart and thus causing less blood flow to the skin. This vayu in the skin also regulates the functions of the sweat glands.

All sorts of inflammation of nerves giving rise to numbness, tingling, pricks of needles in the hands and feet, increased sensitiveness or pains, loss of sensation, trophic and vasomotor changes occurring in one particular part are attributed to (Vat) वात which by its irritation or disordered action *cause* certain molecular changes, which give rise to those sensations given above. Thus the disease neuritis mentioned in Western science is attributed to disordered condition of (Vat) वात in that particular area.

Disorders of special sense such as hearing, smell, taste and vision are attributed to (Pran vayu) प्राणवायु the seat of which is in the brain.

Chapter XI

Ayurvedic Drugs and Their Properties

अघाड़ा (Aghada) is a sedative diuretic, useful against derangements arising from disorders of Kuff in the system for adults. Ashes of (Aghada) आघाड़ा 5 grains.

Juice of Ginger	drachm.
Honey	30 minims

To be taken twice a day. Useful in Cough, Asthma and enlarged spleen in Malaria. Root of this if put at the os, uterus relieves pain at the time of painful menstruation and promotes flow. Chewing of the root relieves toothache and pains in scorpion-bite on application of the root.

अतिविष (Atiwish) Aconite ferrox antiperiodic and useful in fevers. For adults. Powdered Aconite अतिविष (Atwish grs 10)

Aqua ... ... 1 ounce.

Thrice a day

It is also useful in diarrhoea in children

Aconite अतिविष (Atiwish) one grain

(Nagarmotha) नागरमोथा one grain

(Kakarashinghi) काकडशिंगी one grain

Make powder, to be taken twice a day in diarrhoea of children.

Tonic

अतिविष (Atiwish)	1 grain.
नागरमोथा (Nagarmotha)	1 "
काकडशिंगी (Kakarshinghi)	1 "
सागरगोटा (Sagargota)	1 "

Bundook seed make one powder and give in milk.

N.O. Compositac Anacyclus Pyrethrum.

अक्कलकाड़ा (Akkalkara): It has stimulant properties and useful against वात (Vat)

अक्कलकाड़ा (Akkalkara)	... grains ii
Honey	... 3 i—Twice a day, good for

Slammering and tetany.

अगस्था (Agastha) Aperient.

Juice of अगस्था (Agastha) leaves 10 drops in little water is useful in entric fever.

10 to 15 drops of this juice is given as aperient for children in little milk.

N.O. Scitaminace curcuma Amada.

आंबीहळद (Ambe halad) external application reduces inflammation, useful application externally in case so enlarged gland, spleen, liver, allays itching of the skin when applied with कडुजिरे (Kadujeere).

N. O. Anonaceac saraca Indica.

अशोक (Ashok) useful in monorrhagia.

Has astringent properties.

Inner bark of अशोक (Ashok)	one drachm.
Rice water	5 drachms.

Honey. .... 2 drachms—To be taken twice.

आपटा (Apta) useful in painful micturition

Juice of आपटा (Apta) leaves one drachm in one or two ounces of milk. It allays painful micturition and phosphoturia.

N.O. Scilaminaceal Rhizome of Zingeber Official.

आले (Ale) ginger: It is against (Vat) वात.

It has mostly stimulant properties useful in digestion गुलम वायगोला (Gulam waygola) and colic.

Juice of ginger ... one drachm.	useful in indigestion.
Juice of lemon ... two drachms.	
पादेलोन (Padelon) ... 30 grains	

| Juice of ginger ... one drachm. | useful in cough |
| Honey ... ... 2 drachms. | |

Increasing doses of ginger from one drachm to 4 drachms for six days and then decreasing for six days with little milk and rice improves appetite to a great extent.

Juice of ginger one drachm in little sugar stops vomiting and if applied to the sloin stops fainting, external application with little salt is useful in painful joints.

Garlic juice 30 minims.	stimulant.
Juice of ginger 30 minims.	
Water ... 4 drachms.	

Lukewarm juice 5 drops in little milk; stops ear-ache

Myrobalan Embelic.

आंवला (Awala) It is against Pitt and it is diuretic.

| Juice of आंवला one drachm | useful in painful micturition. |
| Honey ... one drachm | |

It is good against आम्लपित्त (Amlapitt)

Juice of आवला 2 drachms.
जिरे ... one drachm
Sugar ... one drachm.
} good against acidity of stomach.

आवलकढी (Anwalkadi), Dried आवला (Awla) in little milk well pounded and applied to the skin is useful in allaying itch and headache.

आस्कंद अश्वगंध (Askand Ashwagandh): These are white sticks obtainable in Indian bazars. It is useful in painful joints.

Root of अश्वगंध (Ashwagandh) powder 10 grains.

Ghee --- --- --- one drachm.

To be taken twice a day.

It is also aphrodisiac when taken with the same dose in cow's milk twice a day or in soup. It is also useful in Leucorrhoea.

आहालीव (Ahaliwa): These are red seeds. They are soaked in 4 ounces of water and given to stop Hiccough. It has sedative properties.

(12) Massas...one...tola...one rupee—180 grains.)

It also produces milk, coconut juice one ounce; warm and put in 3 drachms of (Ahalimb) and stir and put in little sugar. It is also eaten as लाडु (Laddu) N.O. Plantagena seeds of Plantago ovata. इसबगोल (Isabgol). It is against diarrhoea.

10 grains of this is useful against chronic diarrhoea and luecorrhoea.

Isabgol 60 grains to be soaked in four ounces of water to be taken in little sugar. It is also good against arsenical poisoning. It is given with the same dose in curd (दही) Dahi.

इंद्रजव (Indrajaw): These are the seeds of कुडा (Kuda). It is a bazar medicine. Useful in all fevers.

Indrajaw ... 180 grains.
Water ... 1 pint.

Boil to 8th. One ounce to be taken twice a day useful in diarrhoea and fever. One drachm of this infusion with little डिकेमाली (Dikamalee) is given to children for round worms.

| Parched Indrajava | ... grains 40 | To be taken every four hours useful in colic. |
| पादेलोन (Padelon) (Black salt) | ... grains 10 | |

ईडालिंबु (Idalimbu) Citrin useful against copper poisoning.

उपलसरी (Upalsari), अनंतमुल (Anantmul)
It is alternative.

उपलसरी (Upalsari) ... 3 tolas or one ounce.
Water ... 4 pints.

Make decoction to 1/8th. one ounce of this decoction to be taken twice a day with little sugar. In the same dose it is also diuretic.

उपलसरी (Upalsari) ... one sola or 160 grs.
हिरडेदल (Hirdedal) ... ... -do- ... -do- ...
गोखरू (Gokhru) ... ... -do- ... -do- ...

Water half seer or 16 ounces, decoction to 1/4th. one ounce twice a day useful tonic to allay irritation in gonorrhoea.

डंबर (Umber) Counter irritant for enlargement and inflamed glands.

3 drops of this juice in little *Sugar* 2 grs. is good in diarrhoea of children. The bark of this is raw fruit after macerating it in little water allays thirst and external application of this over the head is good in case of whooping cough in children. Bark of Umber tree 4 tollas or one ounce, water 2½ pint decoction to 1/8th one ounce twice a day used in syphilis.

The same decoction has healing properties in wounds.

ऊद (Ood) antiseptic and deodorant. It is to be pounded in little liquor and applied in the wound, it stops bleeding. It is also good in menorrhagia by putting powdered ऊद (Ood) in little lint at the os-uterus sugar cane. It is diuretic. It is against Pitt and useful in कामीला (Kamila) jaundice.

N. O. Convolvulaceal Recinis communis.

एरंड (Arand) Castor oil plant. ... one tola or 180 grains.

Root एरंड (Arand)

Water ... ... 16 ounces.

Make decoction to 1/8th. Honey 2 drachms, one ounce to be taken twice a day acts as aperient. It is antiphlogestic, Poultice of castor oil leaves and seeds useful in inflamed and painful joints and mastitis. It also diminishes the flow of milk by poulticing.

Juice of castor oil plant leaves 2 drachms.

Sugar 4 drachms and water one ounce useful in jaundice and enlarged spleen.

Castor oil. Aperient, in indigestion, colic. If you take little whey, throughout and then drink castor oil you feel no taste. External application of this oil (massaging) and daily aperient reduces the size.

ओवा (Owa), अजमोदा (Ajmoda) useful in indigestion and aperient and appetizer against worms.

पादेलोन (Padelon) ...   grs. x.
ओंवा (Owa) ...   grs. x.

To be given every day at night time stops worms. It promotes digestion of wheat flour, milk by mixing it a little. It is anti-diuretic.

ओंवा (Owa) ...   grs. x
गुळ (Gul) ...   grs. x.

Make pill to be taken twice a day. It is also against iructation. External application relieves pain and toothache and against perspiration in fevers.

किरमणी ओवा (Kermani Owa). It is useful in indigestion colic. It is very good against worms.

किरमणी ओवा (Kermani Owa)	...	grs. v
वावर्डींग (Bawding)	... ...	grs. v
गुळ (Gul)	...	grs. x

Given at night time. It destroys the worms.

खुरासनी आवा (Khurasani Owa). It produces sleep.

खुरासनी ओवा (Khurasani Owa) grs x in little water.

कचरा (Kachra). These are black round roots of the tree called Kachra.

कचरा (Kachra). It is strengthening food.

कचरा (Kachra) divested of its outer covering is well pounded and boiled in milk and sugar.

कचरा (Kachra)	...	one tola i.e. 180 grains.
Milk	...	8 ounce.
Sugar	...	one ounce

Alkaloid like गुळबेल सत्व (Gulbel satva) is also taken out of the bark after macerating it in water. It acts as tonic.

कचोरा (Kachora): It is called शढी (Shatti). It is very good in fever especially malarial.

| कचोरा (Kachora) | ... | one tola or 180 grains. |
| Water | ... | 16 ounces. |

Boil to 1/8th. One ounce to be taken twice a day. It is appetiser in 10 grain doses and stops vomiting and hiccough if infusion is taken in drops. It is against Pitt.

Powdered कचोरा (Kachora) 2 grains
Honey ...   ...   30 drops

It is against worms in children. It also increases the growth of the hair on external application.

कडु कवठी (Kadukawathe): It is called चलमोगरा (Chalmogra) in Bengali useful in skin diseases. Oil of this 2 ounces and sandal oil 2 ounces to be applied over the skin and 5 drops of the oil in 2 ounces of milk to be taken once a day. Diet should be milk and rice and no salt.

कडुजिरे (Kadujire): It is against cough.

कडुजिरे (Kadujire) 2 grains in little honey is given against cough in children.

कडुजिरे (Kadu jire)	100 grains
Sugar	one ounce
Water	one pint.

Boil to 1/8th, one tea spoonful to be given and the same when applied mixed with little milk and Tilli oil allays itching.

कोड़ (Kod) *Leucoderma*.

कडुजिरे (Kadu jire)	4 drachms
हरताल (Hartal)	4 drachms
हिरडा (Hirda)	" -do-
बेहडा (Behda)	" -do-
आंवला (Awla)	" -do-

Should be well pounded in 4 ounces of cow's urine and applied.

कडुनिंब (Kadunimb): Anti periodic in fevers.

कडुनिंब (Kadunimb)	4 ozs.
कुटकी (Kutki)	"
काडे चिरायति (Kade chirayati)	"
गुळबेल (Gulbel)	"
अतिविष (Ativish)	"

Water 4 seers. Boil to 1/8th. One ounce is to be taken in little honey twice a day.

Inner bark-grs. X, sulphur grs. X, sugar 2 drachms twice a day useful in syphilis.

Flowers of this tree are aperient, dried flowers-grs. X.

कमल (Kamal) Lotus—It is good in heart diseases, 10 grains or 3 masas of dried lotus, one drachm of honey, 2 drachms butter and little sugar allays palpitation.

It is against Pitt. Decoction of निलोफर (Nilofar) (blue lotus) two drachms and 8 ounces of water to boil 1/8th. One ounce twice a day useful in fever, chronic phthisis, diarrhoea, menorrhagia.

करंज (Karanj) oil of this is beneficial in all skin diseases and application of seeds reduces inflammation of lymphatic glands and useful in fistula in ano.

करडयी (Kardai) seeds 5 drachms, to be well pounded in 8 ounces of milk is useful in scanty micturition.

कस्तुरी (Kasturi) Musk stimulent.

Dried secretion from the preputial follicles of moscus moskiferrous.

1 grain in betal leaves twice a day is good in cyncopy and heart failure. It is also aphrodisiac.

1 grain mixed with 3 grains of गुळबेल सत्व (Gulbel-Satv) is useful in fevers.

कपिला (Kapila): It is obtainable in bazar, it is an aperient and against worms. 2 grs. in little milk in chidren produces copious motions.

काकड़ शिङ्गी (Kakad Shingi): It is good against cough in children. बालघुटी (Balghuti) consists of अतिविष, नागरमोथा and काकड़ शिङ्गी (Atiwish, Nagarmotha and Kakar Shingi) one grain each, acts as a tonic and against fever in children. कांचन (Kanchan): It is good against enlarged glands. Bark 4 drachms in eight ounces of water boil to 1/8th one ounce to be taken twice a day. Bark is also applied externally to the glands.

कात (Kat) Catechu good in diarrhoea has astringent properties. It is against frequent micturition useful in chronic ulcers and inflammation 10 grains in 4 ounce of water early in the morning reduces obesity.

कात गोली (Kat goli) consists of कात, जायफल, चंदन, लवंग, कंकोल बेलदोड़े (Kat, Jayfaul, Chandan, Long, Kankol Beldode) in equal parts with little musk and sarsafron to be put in केवडा (Kewda) leaves for seven days one grain of this in betal leaves increases appetite and improves voice.

कांदा (Kanda) onion. They are either red or white aperient and against piles and indigestion one drachm of juice mixed with one drachm of ginger is very beneficial for indigestion, one drachm of juice is also good in early diarrhoea of cholera. One drachm of juice should be taken every third hour. It produces sleep. It acts as stimulant like ammonia if given to smell, good in fainting, acts as poultice against inflammation.

कापुस (Kapus) cotton used in external application as fomentation against inflammation. Clean cotton is soaked in water about an hour and then fried in ghee and then applied over the inflammant part. Smoke of cotton in the nose stops bleeding.

कपुर (Kapur) Camphor: It is diaphoretic.

5 grains in little water and local anaesthetic and against worms and colic. It has also stimulant properties.

4 grains at night time in little water stops night emissions. External application over the womb in little ghee stops pains.

Camphor 2 grains and asafoetida 2 grains is good in Asthma and palpitation. Camphor one drachm in coconut oil one ounce is useful in painful joints and in enlarged glands.

Camphor 6 grains, musk 2 grains is useful in causing labour pains. It is given in betal leaves. Useful in bedsores camphor 10 grains and catachu 10 grains.

कार्लें (Karle): It is useful against cough in children and aperient. 40 minims of juice is useful against worms.

गेरू (Geru): It is tonic and astringent and useful in mouth diseases. Application of this in little milk is useful in sore-eyes.

गेरू (Geru): 10 grains and ginger 10 grains in little milk and sugar is useful in acid dyspepsia.

Chiretta किरायीत (Kirayati): It is tonic antiperiodic and used in malarial fever as infusion.

कुडा (Kuda). It is useful in mucoid diarrhoea and against worms and astringent. Bark 15 grains in little whey mixed with one grain of asafoetida and two grains of Dikemali twice a day kills worms.

Bark 4 ounces to be well pounded in 2 pints of water and boil to one half pint in old गुळ (Gul) 8 ounces and then mixed with 20 grains each of ginger myrrh, Pipeli, Hirada, Awala, Indrajawa, Wawding and Wala, one drachm each in powder and mixed one ounce of honey. It acts well in diarrhoea.

कुठकी (Kutki). It is good against malaria. 5 grains in gum 5 grains. It is aperient and useful in hiccough. Decoction of one tola of this in one pound of water boil to 1/8th is also useful in jaundice.

Sarsafron केशर (Kesar): It is stomachic, stimulent. Camphor केशर (Keshar) and sandalwood is good as external application in headache.

Sarsafron grains 2, camphor grains. V is good to promote uterine flow.

Plantain tree केळ (Kel).

Fruit acts as tonic and astringent while केळफुल (Kelful) is appetiser and is against worms.

One drachm juice of this tree is good in dysentery and promotes flow of urine and useful in epistaxis used also as external application in little water to wash ulcers and in washing ears and in skin diseases, useful in piles.

Juice of this tree is allowed to remain in open vessel for 2 days. The precipitate is taken out and dried. 5 grains of this in little water is useful in dropsy and scanty micturition.

Korfud कोरफ (Korfud): It is stimulant and appetiser and aperient and against cough in children. Juice of कोरफड (Korfud) leaves one drachm in little milk early in the morning is appetiser. Korfud juice one drachm.

नवसागर (Nowsagar): Ammonium chloride grs. V.

Common salt. grs. V.

Useful in enlarged liver and spleen and in dropsy. External application of कोरफड, मंजिष्ट (Korfud, Manjist) and हळद (Halad) is useful in skin diseases and epistaxis. It is astringent, external application of कोरफड (Korfud) with the same quantity of allum and 5 grains of opium subdues inflammation in sore-eyes and reduces the inflammation in piles.

कालबोल (Kalabol) (Mussabar): An exernal application reduces inflammation. Famous Kumari Asav contains Korpud कोरफड (Korfud).

It is extensively used in promoting stools in new born children by giving it in 2 grain doses in 3 drops of ghee and 2 drops of honey.

कंकेल (Kankol): It is against Pitt and useful in indigestion, externally used to allay itching due to indigestion. It has astringent properties. Oil of this is externally used in fissures in the hands and feet.

कोहला (Kohla): It is beneficial in diseases arising from blood. Juice of this 2 drachms in little sugar stops bleeding. It is astringent and used in Haemoptysis and used also in tonic in कोहलेपाक (Kohlepak).

कंकोल (Kankol): It is diuretic.

2 grains of this sandalwood grs. V in little sugar produces free flow of urine, used also in gonorrhoea. It is called शितलाचिनी कोष्ट (Shitlachini koshta). It is against Kuff and sedative acts against Vat and Pitt. It is also used against Asthma and Dysmenorrhoea.

कोष्ट (Koshta) grs. VI, camphor grains 10 in little honey every two hours stops the pain.

कोष्ट (Koshta) grs iii, honey one drachm useful in cough.

खसखस (Khaskhas) poppy seeds, tonic, astringent, in diarrhoea. Poppy heads are useful in fomentations.

खजुर (Khajoor) Dates: It is tonic and against Pitt and against enlargement.

खडु (Khadu) chalk. It is against wat and sedative chalk grs. x in one ounce of milk and little sugar stops burning in acidity, to be taken after food. Astringent in diarrhoea when given in honey.

Soothes cough in a grain dose in children.

Chalk one ounce and tilli oil 2 (ounces) used as external application in ulcers.

कौडल (Kowdal) cathartic purgative used in dropsy. Contents of fruit 5 grains, rock salt 10 grains, black salt पादेलोन (Padelon) grs.x used in enlarged liver.

खारीक (Kharik): Astringent and tonic, well pounded in ghee is used as tonic.

गुगुल (Guggul): It is alterative and against Vat.

Decoction of गुळबेल (Gulbel) and ginger 1 dr. boil to 1/8th put in 10 grs. of guggul one ounce twice a day allays pains in the joints and muscles.

हिरडा (Hirda)	1 oz.
बेहडा (Behada)	1 oz.
Awala	1 oz.
Water	2 pints. 40 ounce

Boil to 1/2, put in गुगुल (Guggul) 4 drachms and boil and take it out and dry, 10 grs of this is taken in little honey and ghee acts as a tonic and against piles when taken in little hot water, external application over the chest stops hiccough and useful in skin diseases.

खैर (Khair): It is sedative and blood purifier and astringent decoction of two ounces in two pints of water is used as month wash in inflammed gums. It is used in diarrhoea and cough.

गुलबेल (Gulbel): It is alterative. Tonic and bitter, extensively used in malarial fevers and enlarged spleen.

गुलबेल	(Gulbel)	1 oz.	Boil to 1/2 half, one ounce twice a day useful in malarial fevers and dyspepsia.
पित्तफपडा	(Pittkapda)	1 oz.	
नागरमोथा	(Nagarmotha)	1 oz.	
Chiretta		1 oz.	
Water		32 ozs.	

गुलबेल सत्व (Gulbel satwa) 3 to 5 grs. useful in chronic fevers when taken in little ghee and honey.

गेलफल (Gelphal): It is an emetic. Bark of the fruit 4 drachm and an ounce of water, one ounce to be taken early in the morning. It is against worms, use 3 grs. of the powdered fruit.

गोखरू (Gokhru): It is diuretic. 1 ounce of Gokhru and water 16 ounces, boil to 1/8th, one ounce to be taken twice a day.

गोखरू	(Gokhru)	2 drachms	Tonic against night emissions.
आवलकढी	(Anwalkati)	2 "	
गुलबेल	(Gulbel)	2 "	
Milk		2 ounces	

In little milk in 10 grs doses stops leucorrhoeal discharges in women.

गोपीचंदन (Gopichandan) sedative and astringent, useful in epistaxis 3 gr. doses in little honey in Haemoptysis stops menorrhagia on external application at the os-uterus.

गोरोचन (Gorochan): It is the cow's bile used in measles in two gr, doses in little milk and also in Typhoid fever when eruptions are absent. Used in Tetany with little बेखंड (Bhekhand) Sulphur गंधक (Gandhak) 10 grs in one plantain is good in piles. It is also a purgative. Sulphur 2 drachms, tilli-oil one ounce coconut oil 4 drachms to be heated and allowed to cool, use as external application in case of scabies and skin diseases.

Tamarind चिंच (Chinch): It is acid, aperient used in some cases of dyspepsia. It stops vomiting and colic in 2 grain doses of the ash. Its seeds are used in whooping cough among children by external application on the head.

गोरखचिंच (Gorakhchinch) is useful in आल्मपित्त (Amalpit), acid dyspepsia and diarrhoea 20 grains in whey thrice a day.

It is used in cholera as follows: विसुचिका (Vishuchika) Old Tamarind one ounce, garlic soaked in whey 4 drachms and marking nut one, to be well pounded and make 5 grains pill to be given every 15 minutes in one drachm juice of onions.

चित्रक (Chitrak): It is cathartic, purgative and useful in dyspepsia.

Chittrak	10 grs.	
वावडींग (Wavding)	20 grs.	5 grains to be taken in one drachm of honey.
नागरमोथा (Nagarmotha)	20 grs.	

Used also in skin diseases as external application.

It is also used in enlargements of liver and spleen. It is also used in leuco derma. Chittrak one drachm well rubbed in one ounce of milk and when rubbed in liquor is useful in painful joints and enlarged glands.

Lime चुना (Chuna) antacid useful in acid dyspepsia. Lime water two drachms and 4 ounces milk, useful in hiccough when mixed with Anisi oil 2 minims. It is used externally in enlargement of glands. Internally lime water and milk as given above used in guinea-worm. Two drachms lime water and 3 ounces of Til oil is used in burns and in skin diseases and in syphilis to improve ulcers.

Lime water 8 ounces and mercuric-perchloride 3 grains useful in syphilitic ulcers. In mad dog bite external application of lime acts as antiseptic and caustic.

हरताल ((Hartal): Arsenic sulphide 160 grains and 12 drachms of चुना (Chuna) destroy hair.

चोपचिनी (Chopchini) tonic. It is a bazar medicine aperient.

चोपचिनी (Chopchini) 30 grains.

Ginger juice one drachm acts as purgative.

चोपचिनी (Chopchini) 20 grains. ⎤ useful in syphilitic
Decoction of Indian Sarsaparilla. ⎦ ulcers.

अनंतमुल (Anantmul) 6 drachms, in one seer of water boil to 1/8th Chopchini 160 grains.

Ghee 2 drachms, make 20 grains pills twice a day useful in night emiissions.

Weak Decoction is diaphoretic.

चंदन (Chandan) sandalwood it is used to reduce inflammation externally.

चंदन (Chandan) 4 drachms, water 16 ounces boil to 1/8th. It is good in fevers. Tonic 3 grains of चंदन (Chandan) in little ghee acts as stimulant to the heart. It is also diuretic as decoction. Extensively used in gonorrhoea.

कंकोल ((Kankol) 160 grains, बंशलोचन (Banslochan) 160 grs., sandalwood oil 30 minims. make 3 grs, pills good in gonorrhoea.

जटामासी (Jatamansi): It is a bazar medicine.

जटामासी (Jatamansi) grs. x बेखंड (Bekhand) grs.x, Honey drs, 2 useful in hysteria.

जटामासी (Jatamansi) one ounce, दशमुल (Dashamul) one ounce, water one seer, boil to 1/8th one ounce twice a day. It is useful as a blood purifier. It increases the hair growth on external application.

जवस (Jawas) Linseed: It is demulcent.

जवस (Jawas) 4 drachms, ज्येत्रमध (Jaitramadh) one dr., well pounded and boiled in water one seer allays painful urination. Useful as poultice in fevers in acute bronchitis, pneumonia used to ripen boils by poulticing.

जाई (Jai): Good as mouth wash.

हिरडा, (Hirda,) बेहडा, (Behda), आवला, (Awla), दारू (Daru), हलद (Halad) and leaves of Jai in equal parts and one seer water boil to 1/6th good as mouth wash. Application of pounded leaves cures ulcers.

जांबुल (Jambul) Tree: It is digestive, stops diarrhoea. Bark of Jambul tree 10 drachms in one seer of water boil to 1/6th. One ounce of this is taken with little honey twice a day, useful in diarrhoea and also in leucorrhoea. Jambul juice is good in cholera, diabetis enlarged spleen and colic.

Jambul seeds 45 grs 4 times a day is useful in reducing sugar in diabetes. It is to be taken in hot water. It is required to be taken for two months. Decoction is also used as mouth wash. External application of the seed cures acne.

जायफल (Jaifal): It is astringent used in cholera. 10 grains every two hours in little Gur (गुल) (Gul) stops diarrhoea. It also removes foul smell from the mouth, used as external application in headache. Application to the eyes produce sleep.

जायपत्री (Jaipatri): It is stimulant and used as musk कस्तूरी (Kasturi), जासवंद (Jasvand). Five young flowers of white जासवंद (Jasvand) should be fried in ghee and add little sugar. One to be taken early in the morning, stops leucorrhoea, useful in avoiding abortion. It increases the growth of hair. Juice of Jasvand flower is used for this purpose on the hairs to promote hair growth.

Oil is used as hair restorer.

जिरें (Jeere): It stops diarrhoea.

जिरे (Jeere) 60 grs, बावर्डींग (Wawding) 60 grs. stops, hiccough and is against worms.

खंबायतीजिरा (Khambaiti jeera) is good in diarrhoea.

जेष्टमध (Jaisht madh): It is tonic. 60 grs. in little honey is to be taken twice a day. Decoction of ज्येष्टमध (Jaisht madh) zii and in 16 ounces of water, boil to 1/8th useful in curing ulcers in the mouth, clears the voice in 3 grs. doses mixed with 3 grs. of मिरे (Meere).

अडुलसा (Adulsa)	60	grs.
जेष्टमध (Jaishtmadh)	160	grs. ro 1 tola.
हिरडे (Hirde)	60	grs.
मनुका (Manuka)	160	grs.

Water 60 seers boil to 1/8th useful to stop bleeding from the chest. It allays cough, thirst, breathlessness and stops bleeding, in bleeding piles in 20 grains doses, in 10 grs doses in 4 ounces of milk it stops scanty and painful micturition.

जेष्टमध (Jaishtmadh) Powder	one tola or 160 grs.
बडीशोप (Badisop)	" "
Sulphur	60 grs.
सोना मखी (Sonamakhi)	30 grs.
Crystallized Sugar	one ounce.

20 grs. of this should be taken at bed time with the water. It acts as aperient and appetiser. It stops menorrhagia. 120 grs ज्येष्टमध (Jaishtmadh) to be rubbed in one ounce milk and mixed with दारूहळद (Daru Halad) 40 grs to be taken twice a day in the morning and evening. It reduces inflammation externally and in skin diseases.

(Jhendu) juice is made out of flowers and mixed with ghee and applied over the bleeding piles. An application as poultice mixed with हळद (Halad) stops pains at the piles.

टाकळा (Takala) externally, leaves well pounded are used in skin diseases. Flowers of Takala 160 grs, mixed in sugar allays painful micturition. It reduces inflammation externally. Application of seeds in Karanj oil and Sulphur cures ring-worm and when mixed with निवडुंग (Niwdung) juice cures all skin diseases.

टाकनखार (Takankhar) sold in bazar as तेलियासुहागी (Teliasohagi), रचौकीसुहागी (Choukisohagi). It is good against cough. 3 grs of burnt Takankhar is useful in whooping cough in children. Ten grs. of burnt Takankhar in betal leaves is useful in fevers. It stops diarrheoea in small dosels. In 20 gr. doses in lemon juice is useful in indigestion, and in little honey is allays pain in dysmenorrhoea. It is Ecbolic in 15 gr doses used externally to promote healing of ulcers and wounds. It is against aconite poisoning.

टेटू (Tetu) bark decoction is diaphoretic.

Tetu bark   6 drachms. } Boil to 1/6th one ounce
Water   16 ounce.   } twice a day.

160 minims. Juice of the bark in little ghee stops diarrhoea. Powdered bark 160 grs.in 3 drs of ghee stops menorrhagia. It is good in piles. Powdered bark 100 grs, ginger 50 grs, Indrajava 50 grs and one drachm of this should be taken in 8 ounce of whey. It is useful in piles. It is also useful in ear-ache.

डामर (Damar) 4 drs in little coconut oil one oz, is useful in eczema.

Pomogranate डाळींब (Dalimb): It is against Pitt, allays thirst and is useful in diarrhoea. Its roots kill worms.

Pomogranate bark 160 grs. वावडींग (Wawding) 6 drs. Indrajava 6 drs, water one seer boil to 1/6th, one ounce twice a day. It is good in indigestion. Powdered bark 100 grs. जायफळ (Jaiful) 40 grs, केशर (Keshar) 20 grs. and Pomagranate juice 2 drs, 30 grs to be taken twice a day. It is good against Jaundice. It is good in consumption when the juice is given in milk. It is good to remove white speckles in the eyes. It improves the voice. It is used also in curing skin eruptions due to spedu on the skin.

डिकेमाली (Dikemali) one grain of डिकेमाली (Dikemali) in little of milk produces stools. It kills worms एलियाबोळ (Aliyabol) and Asafoetida, well rubbed and applied over the stomach removes distention. It is useful in malarial fevers in 10 gr doses. External application cures skin diseases. Ten grs of डिकेमाली (Dikemali) in ginger juice and lemon juice stops colic and useful in indigestion and vomiting. तरवड (Tarwad) bark is tonic, juice stops vomiting. Application of rubbed seeds in water over the granulations is useful. Washing the teeth with Tarwad strengthens them तरवड (Tarwad) tonic 10 grs. of powdered bark in little ghee is given as tonic, powdered seeds in water are used to reduce the granulations in the eyes and ashes are used to strengthen the teeth as dentrifice.

ताक (Tak) butter milk made out of curd after adding water and removing the butter. It is slightly astrigent and appetiser. It is extensively used in cases of piles. It promotes flow of urine and in enlargement of spleen.

According to Ayurveda is harmful in epistaxis and in case of fevers due to injuries. It should always be taken at dinner time. तीळ (Till). It is tonic and food. It is also beneficial in bleeding piles, in 4 drs doses five powders taken with butter. It is also good as antiphlogistic against inflammation, reduces frequency of micturition, relieves stomach ache when taken with little hot water. It has sedative properties when applied to the burns, it promotes the growth of hair.

तिरफळ (Tirphal): These are small fruits like मिरे (Mire). It is also called Tumpal. 10 grs powdered seeds in one dr of ginger juice is good in distention of stomach with colic. It promotes saliva and stops hiccoughs and vomiting. It tetaney with lock jaw given in small doses it is useful in children.

तुरटी (Turti) Allum: It is called फटकरी (Fatkari.) It is put in water and boiled and strained. Alum is precipitated. It is very good against रक्तपित्त (Rakt pitt) and is used in hoemoptysis, epistaxis and rectal bleeding 10 grs, with little honey is given twice a day. It is also used in menorrhagia and bleeding piles mixed with til and butter. It is also applied externally on them. It is astrigent and is used to stop diarrhoea in decoction of वेखंड (Bekhand) 4 drs, eight ounces water, boil to 1-8th and adding one dr. of alum, one ounce to be taken twice a day. It is also given as prophylactic in cholera epidemic 5 grs of alum; 5 grs of catechue and 5 grs. of cinnamon; four times a day. It stops frequency of micturition given with Aniseed in 10 gr doses. It is an excellent medicine in whooping cough of children in 2 gr doses in little honey. It is extensively used in diseases of the eyes and especially in granulations. Put 20 grs of alum in one ounce of water and bathe the eyes with it and rub the granulations. It is also used externally mixed in white of an egg to reduce inflammation in case of injuries to the eyes. For bleeding piles it is an excellent medicine for external use.

मांयफळ (Maefal) one ounce.

Bark of Babool tree	4 drs.
Alum	4 drs.
Water	1 seer.

Boil to 1/2 half and wet a piece of cloth, and put on piles prolapse of rectum and in epistaxis and in bleeding, in injuries, menorrhagia and ulcerations of the mouth, mixed with cocum oil in 20 gr. doses used in fissures of the feet. Alum solution is used in scorpion bite and painful joints externally.

तुलस (Tulas): It is stimulant tonic and antiperiodic. It acts against वात (Vat) and has diaphoretic properties. Extensively used against cold and asthma. Decoction of one ounce of Tulas leaves in 8 ounces of water, boil to 1/8th is good as appetiser twice a day. Juice of Tulasi leaves with little sugar stops Asthmatic fit. One ounce of decoction, mentioned above is given in fevers to promote perspiration and in dry cough. Juice is applied in various skin diseases and in bites from wasp sting. In headache due to Kuff that is to cold dried powdered leaves are used as snuff.

दालचिनी (Dalchini): Cinnamon. It is astringent used in indigestion and colic. Decoction one ounce is used in Influenza.

दालचिनी (Dalchini): 4 drs जेष्टमध (Jaishtmadh) 4 drs, बड़ीशोप (Badisop) 4 drs, crystallised sugar 1 dr, black grapes 1 dr, almonds 5 drs powder and make pills of 5 grs, to be taken 4 times a day useful in dry cough.

दालचिनी (Dalchini) Cardamom seeds four dramchs, बंसलोचन (Banslochan) 8 drs, पिंपली (Pipeli) 2 drs, crystallised sugar 4 drs, make 5 gr pills to be taken 4 times a day. This is called सितोपलाचूर्ण (Sitoplachuran) useful in all cases of indigestion and chronic fevers.

दारूहलद (Daru Halad) Berberry root 1¾.

दारूहलद (Daru Halad) Two tolas or 6 drs, water 16 ounces, boil to 1/8th one ounce twice a day. It acts as quinine. It is also useful in Jaundice when given with आवलकडी (Awalkari). One ounce of decoction is given in enlarged spleen and liver. In 40 gr doses three times a day, it stops menorrhagia.

रसोत (Rasot) is a bazar drug made out of Daruhalad. 20 grs of this in one ounce of rice water with one dr. of crystillised sugar and one dr honey is useful in diarrhoea with blood.

Rasanjan or Rasot 140 grs.

Powdered कडुनिंब (Kadunimb) seeds 10 grs.

Dried grapes 200 grs.

Make 5 gr pills one pill to be taken 4 times a day. It stops blood in bleeding piles.

Grapes मनुका (Manuka) given with rock salt, it is aperient with.

वडीशोप (Badisop): It is used in acidity of stomach. In dry cough with crystallised sugar खड़ीसाखर (Khadisakhar) Tonic in debility after fevers with little milk after food. With rock salt it is useful in jaundice, haemoptysis and epistaxis.

Root of उंबर (Umber) one tola or 160 grs, grapes one ounce, water 8 ounce. Boil to ½ one ounce twice a day. It allays thirst. It is used as Tonic in consumptive cases. It cleans the voice relieves scanty micturition.

मनुका (Manuka) one tola, धमासा (Dhamasa) ½ tola, पुनर्नवा (Punarva ½ tola in one ounce of water boil to 1/8th one ounce twice a day as a diuretic.

उरक्षतक्षय (Urakshatkshay) Haemoptysis in consumption.

मनुका (Manuka) one tola mixed with rice लाही (Lahi) in 4 ounces of water and kept for four hours and then strain, put in ½ tola of crystallized sugar and ghee 10 drops to be taken repeatedly. It is used against giddiness caused by cannabis Indica and भांग (Bhang) grapes five tolas soaked in 2 ounces of water and then strain and put in one dramch of rock salt 10 grs jira, 10 grs. मिरेपुड (Mirepud) powdered myrrh. To be taken twice a day.

द्राक्षारिष्ट (Draksharisht): Tonic and strengthening medicine is used in all kinds of diseases. It is made as follows.

Black grapes 2 lbs add 8 pounds of water strain, put in 2 lbs of cane sugar and one pound of honey, put in two ounces of each powdered Dhayati flowers, कंकोल (Kankol), वाल (Vala), sandalwood चन्दन (Chandan), जायफल (Jaifal) sarsafron लवंग (Lvang), cloves, cardamom seeds, तमालपत्र (Tamalputra) and पिंपली (Pipeli) keep these for one month under the sun in a bottle after thoroughly covering it with earth and cloth 2 drachms of this to be taken in one ounce of water twice a day. It is given in diarrhoea, asthma, cough, vomiting, piles and jaundice and to promote micturition.

देवदार (Devdar) Two tolas in 16 ounces (40 tolas) boil to $\frac{1}{8}$th one ounce to be taken twice a day. Useful as diaphoretic, 10 grs in little honey is beneficial in Rheumatism.

बालंत काढ़ा (Balant kadha): Decoction given during puerperal state.

देवदार (Devdar), वेखंड (Vekhand), सुठ (Sont) ginger, कायफल (Kayphal), नागरमोथा (Nagarmotha), चिर यीत (Chirayeet), हिरडा (Hirda), गोखरू (Gokhru), गुलबेल (Gulvel) Inside of बेलफल (Belphal) fruit शहाजिरे (Shahjira) one tola or 4 drachms each in 16 ounces of water boil to 1/8th, strain in 2 drs of ghee, one dramch of rock salt and strain and 5 grs. of Asafoeitida.

देवदाली (Devdali): It is called पित्तफल (Pittfal) in Bombay, कुकुडबेला (Kukudbela) in Gujarati. Emetic 40 grs of the fruit are soaked in one ounce of water strain. 2 drops are given every five minutes to promote vomiting. Decoction is extensively used in rat poisoning. It is antiphlogistic externally and used in reducing the inflammation of piles. Mixed with रिठा (Ritha) fruits in equal parts it is applied in enlarged glands.

धने (Dhane) Coriander: It is diaphoretic, diuretic and stomachic. Decoction is used in mucous diarrhoea.

कोर्थीबीर (Kothimbir) is applied over the piles. Decoction with जेष्ठमध (Jaishtmadh) is used in cough. It acts as stimulant in weak heart when taken with little sugar.

धभासा (Dhamasa) useful in chronic fevers. Dhamasa 1 dr. with crystallized sugar six drs, in 16 ounces of water, one ounce twice a day. It is diuretic. It is used against renal colic and gravels as diuretic and solvent.

धमासा (Dhamasa) 2drs or 3 masas., Hirdedal 2 drs or 3 masas. Inside of बहावा (Bahawa) 2 drs or 3 masas, गोखरू (Gokhru) 2 drs or 3 masas., water 16 ounces, boil to 1/8th and strain, one ounce to be taken twice a day. One oz of decoction twice a day with grapes is used in cough. Sugar of Dhamasa is obtained in bazar called Turbin. In one grain doses it is used to allay cough in children. It is also used as a poultice externally in inflammations.

धायटी (Dhayati) used in menorrhagia. Powdered धायटी (Dhayati) flower one tola, crystallized sugar one dr in 8 ounces of milk to be taken twice a day, stops also diarrhoea in pregnancy.

नवसागर (Navsagar): Ammonium chloride liquifies the expectoration given generally in cough and bronchitis due to old age diaphoretic in 5 to 8 grs doses in little water. Appetiser 10 grs. नवसागर (Navsagar) and 10 grs पादेलोण (Padelon) in 2 drs. of ginger and lemon juices are good in indigestion and colic.

नवसागर (Navsagar) 10 grs ginger 10 grs mirre and 10 grs pipeli to be taken twice a day, useful in diarrhoea, enlargement of liver and spleen and jaundice.

10 grs of नवसागर पादेलोणा (Navsagar Padelon), black slat 10 grs. Asafoetida 2 grains in ginger and lemon juice is usful in colic and indigestion, externally it is used mixed with liquor to allay inflammation and in painful joints. In abscess of the breast in lactation or inflammation external application of नवसागर (Navsagar) in water is very useful.

नागकेशर ((Nagkeshar) in 10 grs. doses with ghee is useful in piles.

नागरमोथा (Nagarmotha) Decoction of 4 drs. in 16 ounces of water boil to 1/8th allays thirst.

Used in all kinds of fever mixed with पित्तपापड़ा (Pitpapra) in equal parts. Has astringent action in diarrhoea in children.

नागबल्ली (Nagballi) Betal leaf: It is stimulant stomachic used in collapse and fainting 20 drops of the juice. 10 drops are also used in allaying cough. Mixed with ginger juice and two grs. of Asafoetida it promotes appetite. It is externally used in enlarged glands and also as poultice. It clears the voice and dry cough. It has aphrodisiac properties.

Juice mixed with the juice of the root is used externally in poisonous bites and when taken internally in 20 drops doses in little water it is also useful in snake poisoning and as poultice mixed with हळद (Halad) and ghee to promote healing of ulcers.

नारळ (Naral): Coconut good in Haemoptysis tonic. Juice of coconut is good against chronic brochitis. It is very useful in गुलम (Gulam) especially in वात, कफ, गुलम (Wat, Kuff, Gulam) in distention due to dyspepsia and promotes the expulsion of worms.

Coconut ghee is good in hemiplagia. Coconut powdered and mixed with हल्द (Halad) allays inflammation. नारलाचीकवटी (Narlachikwati) outer shell of coconut.

Burnt portion mixed in oil is used in leucoderma and oil extracted from it is useful in skin diseases.

Ashes of the fibrous part of the coconut 1 dr. in little honey stops hiccough and vomiting.

Ghee of coconut is used as cod liver oil.

निर्गुंडी (Nirgundi): It is against वात (Wat)

It reduces inflammation externally. Its leaves are boiled in water and eyes with granular lids are fomented and then washed with cold water. It is also used in Dengu fever by giving steam inhalation of the leaves in water. Its oil is used in painful knee joints oil is extracted from the leaves mixed in mustard oil and 8 times butter milk and then boil and strain.

नीलकमल (Neel Kamal): Blue lotus: It is a heart stimulant and tonic. 20 grs. in little honey is given twice a day. In 10 grs. doses it is used in chronic fevers. The root in 5 gr. doses stops diarrhoea and indigestion. Its seed is called कमल काकड़ी (Kamal kakdi) 10 grs. of this in little honey promotes appetite.

निशोतर (Nishotar) 4 drs.

पिंपड़ी (Pimpri) 4 drs.

खड़ी साखर (Khari sakhar) crystallized sugar 12 drachms, one dr. to be taken before food twice a day. Good in dyspepsia and piles.

निशोतर, गुल्बेल, चिरायति, हिरडा, बेहडा and आवला (Nishotar, Gulbel, Chirayti, Hirda, Behda and Awla) six drachms each in 16 ounces of water boil to 1/8th, one ounce to be taken once a day, for forty days. It stops all kinds of malarial fevers and it is also used externally to reduce inflammations. बावर्डींग, त्रिफला

and गुल (Wavding, Trifala, Gul) one tola each and six tolas of निशोतर गुगुल (Nishotar guggul), 12 tolas make sixty pills. One pill is to be taken twice a day, useful in all kinds of skin diseases.

Papai tree पपायी: It is good against worms, juice 2 drs, honey 2 drs; in hot water promotes the expulsion after taking 2 or 3 days. For a child of 10 years, 10 ms. of juice should be given; externally, it is used in enlarged spleen. It is an appetiser and aperient, externally its juice is used in ring-worm. It promotes menstruation.

परवर (Parwar): It is a bitter tonic.

परिपाठ (Paripath) mixed with हीरेददल (Hireddal) one ounce each and grapes one oz. decoction in equal parts twice a day is given in all eruptive fevers such as Typhoid, measles, etc.

पळस (Padas) (Butea frondosa): Its seeds are called रसपापडी (Ras Papdi) 10 grs. to be given once a day for a day or two. They promote expulsion of worms followed by castor oil. Flowers are diuretic, dried powdered flowers grs. V are useful in chronic fevers and it is a diuretic. Externally powdered flowers are applied over the inflammed womb. Its juice mixed with sugar and alum is tonic and strengthening. It is aphrodisiac. Its leaves are used externally to reduce inflammation of the boils. पलस (Palas), रसांजन (Rasanjan) and allum to be well rubbed in rose water and applied to the granulations. Ashes of पलस (Palas) tree after repeated washing in 10 grs. doses acts against cough with Ammonium chloride.

पारिजातक (Parijatak): It is against malaria.

Juice of पारिजातक (Parijatak) leaves 30 ms. mixed in one drachm of ginger juice and in one ounce of hot water to be given twice a day.

पिंपली (Pipeli): It is stimulant. Decoction is used against cough. 10 grs. of Pipeli with 10 grs. of black salt in butter milk should be taken every day in indigestion. वंशलोचन (Vanshlochan) 2 drs, पिंपली (Pipeli) 2 drs, cardamom seeds 2 drs, 10 grs of this to be taken twice a day. It is digestive. पिंपलीपाक (Pipelipak) 4 tolas of pipeli are boiled in 16 ounces of milk till dried and mixed with sugar.

Decoction of पिंपळी, Pipeli and ginger in 16 ounces of water boil to 1/8th. One ounce to be taken with little milk.

पिंपळी रसायन is used in dropsy.

पिंपळ मुल Pipeli mool: It acts like Pipeli. It is principally given to promote sleep. 10 grs. of this powdered root is mixed with गुळ gud. (molasi). 3 grs. of this is to be taken 5 times a day.

पिंपळ Pipel tree: It is called बोधी Bodhi tree in Sanskrit. Its bark is astringent and is used externally to reduce inflammation.

पुदीना (Pudina): It is digestive.

पुनर्नवा (Punarnava). It is diuretic externally, it reduces inflammation, it is used in dropsy as decoction. It is aperient पुनर्नवा Punarnava 2 drs., बाळहिरडे Bal Hirde 2 drs दारूहडद Daru Haradh one d., गुळबेल Gulbale 1 dr., कडुब्रन्दावन Kadu verandawan 1dr. Nisothar one dr., castrol oil root, एरंडमुल Arandmool 1dr. in 16 ounce of water boil to 1/8th ointment of this reduces the granulations of the eyes. पुनर्नवा Punarnava is called पाठरीवसु Patharivasu.

The root is generally used.

बडीशोप Badishope: It is against वात Vat. It is appetiser in 10 grains doses in little honey in the morning. 10 grs.

पादेलोणा Padhelon early in the morning is given in indigestion.

Badishope grs. x and 10 grains Padhalon in stomach colic, decoction of 6 drs, in 16 ounces of water boil to 1/8th one ounce twice a day is useful in fevers and to allay thirst and vomiting and acid dyspepsia.

बाडीशोप Badishope 6 drs, and 4 drs. Khaskhas, Poppy seeds and 16 ounces of water, decoction to 1/8th, one ounce twice a day useful in diarrhoea.

बडीशोप Badishope one ounce, जिरा one dr., one dr. cinnamon and 10 grs. ginger, water 16 ounces. Boil to 1/8th. One ounce twice a day is useful in promoting appetite.

Externally it is applied over the head for headache.

बकुल Bakul powdered bark in 16 ounces of water. Externally it is used as astringent to reduce inflammation. Bakul flowers are diuretic. Infusion of Bakul flowers (40) in 16 ounces of water allays painful micturition in stones of the bladder and dissolves the stone to some extent.

बदाम (Badam) Almonds: It is tonic. Oil is very useful in ear-ache and on the bite of गोम Gom Ash is used as dentrifice.

बाभुळ Babool: Infusion of the leaves is used as mouth wash. Juice one dr. stops diarrhoea given with खडीसाखर Khari Sakhar, crystallized sugar. Gum is tonic.

देवबाभुळ Devbaphul.

Infusion of the flowers promotes perspiration, especially given in typhoid fevers.

Devbaphul flowers 3 drs. in 16 ounces of water boil to 1/8th one ounce twice a day, given in mad dog poisoning.

बावच्यी Bawchi: It is alterative, and also used in Leucoderma.

Powdered Bawchi seeds one ounce prepared sulphur 2 drs dry and applied over the part washing it with carbolic soap.

Sulphur is to be put in covered cloth and suspended in a pot and immersed in lime water and boil for an hour.

बहावा Bahawa: It is called in Bombay गरमाल्याचागोल Garmalyachagol बहावा Bahawa 1 oz, हिरदेदल Hirdedal 6 drs., grapes dried one ounce water, 16 ounces boil to 1/8th and strain useful in epistaxis, piles, and in scantly micturition. It is good aperient in fevers, externally it reduces the inflammation.

बांगडखार Bangdakhar : It is appetiser.

15 grs. is taken in little water relieves the distension of the stomach. Bangdakhar grs. xx, हिरडेदल Hirdedal one drachm., Bahawa 3 drs., water 16 ounces, boil to 1/8th. One ounce twice a day, useful in stomach colic.

80 totals make one seer.

वालंत शोप (Balant shope): It is digestive. 2 drs. should be taken every day, by a woman in a puerperal state, produces good flow of milk. It is also aperient used in stomach colic.

बीबा (Beeba): Marking nut.

बिब्याचेशेवते (Bibyacheshevate) 5 drops in 4 ounces of milk kills worms.

Externally it is used as counter-irritant. Five marking nuts should be punctured with needle and put in ½ seer of water in a tinned vessel boil to 1/8th and mixed with twice the quantity of milk. It is called भल्लातक (Bhallatak) milk is useful in piles due to Vat. It is useful in dyspepsia.

5 marking nuts and 3 drs of बेलफल (Belfal) boil in 16 ounces of water in tinned vessel, to 1/8th and strain and then add equal quantity of milk, useful in मेह (Meh), excessive micturition and in कुष्ठ (Kusht, Skin diseases: Diet—rice and milk. Externally it is used in enlarged glands, oil is extracted as follows:

Put in marking nuts in an earthen pot with a small hole in the centre and put it on a small vessel on the ground and then heat oil falls down in the vessel.

बिरोजा, गंधाविरोजा (Biroza, Ghandha biroza).

20 grs in crystallized sugar is useful in piles, useful in gonorrhoea when taken with milk and crystallized sugar. It is also diuretic. Externally it is used to reduce inflammation. It acts as sticking plaster. External application on the chest reduces cough in children and in Influenza. It promotes the growth of hair when applied to the head. It is also useful in enlarged scrotum due to injury.

बेल (Bel) unripe fruit. 30 grs of dry Bel-phal with little sugar stops diarrhoea.

Ripe fruit is sweet and aperient stops blood in stools. Inside of the Bel धने, सुंठ, नागरमोथा, अनिविष (Dhane, Soonth, Nagarmotha, Atiwish) 50 grs. each and water 16 ounces. Boil to 1/8th one ounce to be taken twice a day. Good in diarrhaea. 30 grs. Bel-phal, ginger 10 grs. stops frequency of desire to go to stools. बेलफल (Bel-phal), Indrajaw and bark of कुड़ा (Kura) 20 grs. each relieves distension of stomach and increases appetite given in small doses in consumption. Decoction of the root of the tree.

Root of the tree 4 drs. water 16 ounces boil to ½.

Good in typhoid fever to produce perspiration, allays palpitation. Externally it is used to reduce inflammation. Bol बोल one is black called बालंतबोल (Balantbol) and the other हिराबोल (Hira Bol). बालंतबोल (Balantbol) 6 grs. and 1 gr. opium, make pill of one grain. One grain pill to be given once a day in the puerperal condition.

बालंतबोल (Balantbol) 2 grs and डिकेमाली (Dikemali) 2 grains, Asafoetida 2 grains make six pills. One pill to be given each in the morning and evening in little milk useful in enlarged spleen and to kill worms in children. कालाबोल (Kala Bol) acts on repetition as aperient. So requires to be given less and less. It is applied externally in children in distension of stomach.

Black कालाबोल (Kalabol) 2 grains ⎤
Red बोळ Bol -do- 2 grains ⎦ Twice a day

हिराकस Hirakas Ferri sulph 2 grs ⎫ Promotes menstrual
Sugar गुळ Gul 4 grains ⎭

बोर (Bor) Demulcent and sedative and diaphoretic.

Rubbing of the seed in water then applying to the sore eyes, reduces inflammation and granulations.

ब्राम्ही (Bramhi): It is extensively used in Tetanus tetanic convulsions and epilepsy.

Juice of the green leaves is rubbed with वेखंड Bekhand with little Tilly oil is rubbed over the head.

ब्राम्ही Brahmi Juice 3 drs.

वेखंड Bekhand 20 grs.

Tilly oil 1 ounce.

To be rubbed over the head. It is also diuretic and used in syphilis. Brahmi juice one dr. mixed with two drs. of cow's ghee and one dr. of honey is given twice a day for 2 or 3 months.

भारंगमुळ (Bharangmul): It is extensively used in Asthma. 20 grs. of the powdered rood is given with little honey in

Asthma, mixed with 10 grs. of Pipeli it is used in Hiccough.

In कफज्वर Kuffjwar when there is no thirst or appetite body is heavy and no perspiration.

Decoction of this 6 massas about 2 drs. in 16 ounces of water boil to 1/8th. One ounce twice a day is very useful.

भुयीमुंग (Bhuimung) Groundnut: It is aperient. Powdered in small quantity it is given to children as tonic. It is given internally in piles. Oil is rubbed to the skin in case of children. It acts as cod liver oil. Powdered ground nut 2 drs. mixed with sugar is given as tonic.

मिरची (Mirchi Powdered) मिरची (Mirchi) 2 grs. in little गुळ (Guda) is given in stomach-ache with acidity.

मिरची (Mirchi) grs. 2, lime grs. 2, onion juice ms. 30, one small tea spoon ful make one pill, useful in cholera. When appetite is lost owing to drinking 2 grs. taken early in the morning promotes appetite.

मिरे (Mire): It is a stomachic and relieves cough.

Powdered mire one drachm, ginger juice one dr. (one small teaspoonfull), lemon juice one dr. To relieve stomach ache. It is used also against worms in small quantities. It acts very well against malaria.

Juice of तुलसी (Tulsi) leaves 2 drs. or two teaspoonfull (11) Eleven powdered मिरे (Mire) twice a day.

मिरे (Mire) 5 tolas, and 16 ounces of water boil to 1/8th To be taken for 7 days. It is also taken along with whey in case of piles. It promotes scanty menstruation. Decoction is used as mouth wash to relieve dental pain.

मीठ (Meeth) Salt: It is stomachic. It liquifies the sputum in children,. grs. 2. are put in teaspoon full of water and repeatedly given. It is also given in stomach-ache due to indigestion in ginger and lemon juice. Externally, it is used against wasp stings. It is germicide. It destroys lice in the hair. It is also emetic. Externally it is applied to relieve headache and jaundice. It also reduces inflammation externally. It also blackens the hair.

मका (Maka) one tola, mire powder 4 tolas, crystallized sugar one tola to be taken early in the morning. Useful in jaundice. Maka oil is used as hair restorer. It is extensively used in obesity with enlarged glands. Rubbed all over the skin.

Earth माटी (Mati) is used as external application in case of burns and wasp bites to relieve pain.

Honey (Medha): Aperient and as mouth wash mixed with water mixed with lime in equal parts, it is used to reduce inflamed glands.

मयफल (Mayphal): It is astringent, used in diarrhoea in children and in menorrhagia and piles.

Powdered मायफल (Mayphal) is put in clean cloth and put at the ox externally it is applied to the piles.

Powdered with Alum it is used as dentifrice to stop bleeding from the gums and teeth. In diarrhoea of children it is rubbed in honey in small quantity and given three times a day.

मालकंगनी (Malkangni.)

Its oil is used externally for painful joints and in hemiplagia in ulcers in skin diseases. Its seeds are rubbed in honey and applied to the piles.

Malkangni seed one, ginger one grs, owa 5 grs, one powder

to be given twice a day in Rheumatic affections of joints and in scanty menstruation.

मुरडशेंग (Muradsheng): It is astringent. Rubbed in little milk it is given in children to stop diarrhoea and put in the ear to stop suppuration.

मुला (Mula) Radish Juice three tolas is taken internally in case of piles. It is stomachic externally it is applied to the piles.

मुसली (Musali): It is tonic.

Powdered white मुसली (Musali) 12 drachms, Almonds 2 drachms to be boiled in 8 ounces of milk and then mixed with one tola of ghee and little sugar taken twice a day.

मोम (Mom) Wax: It is white or yellow.

Wax one ounce, camphor 4 drs., शेंदुर (Shendur) 40 grs., राळ (Ral) 4 drs, are to be boiled in oil and this ointment is applied externally for ulcers and wounds.

मेंदी (Mendi), It is sedative.

Juice one tola mixed in 4 ounces of milk relieves burning sensation in the stomach. In two drops doses it is given to relieve scanty menstruation. It is also useful in diarrhoea with passage of blood mixed with ghee and जीरा (Jeera). It is very useful in diarrhoea after small-pox, measles etc.

Juice 3 drs. in 8 ounces of milk taken a day or two before menstrual period promotes the flow. It also liquifies the sputum in small doses. Juice has emetic properties. It is required to be given diluted in milk and taken in small quantities.

मेंदी (Mendi) bark two tolas, कटुकी (Katuki) one tola, black grapes कार्लोद्राक्षे (Kalidrakshe) one tola, हिरडेदळ (Hirdedal)

½ tola. Water 16 ounce; boil to 1/8th. One ounce twice a day. Useful in jaundice.

Decoction of मेंदी (Mendi) bark one ounce of water is useful against पित्तज्वर (Pitt jwar).

In chronic fevers due to malaria with enlarged spleen decoction is given as follows:

Bark two tolas, Triphala half tola, Wawding one tola, water 16 ounces, boil to 1/8th, one ounce twice a day. Externally it is used against scabies, ringworm, and eczema.

Decoction of 4 tolas of मेंदी (Mendi) flowers in 16 ounces of water boil to 1/8th one ounce of this is mixed in little milk and taken relieves headache.

It is also externally applied to relieve burning sensation of the hands and feet and in diseases of the nails. It also increases the growth of the hair. The oil is used for this purpose. It is good against कुष्ट (Kusht).

मेथी (Methi) externally it is used to reduce inflammation. It is tonic and given in cases of debility.

मैदा-लकड़ी (Maida lakdi) externally it used to reduce inflammation.

हळद, रक्तचंदन (Halad, Raktachandan) Red sandalwood, marking nut बिबाधूप, गुग्गुल, मैदालकड़ी (Bibadhup, Guggul, Maidalakri) mixed together and boiled four drams each and applied externally to reduce inflammation.

मोचरस (Mochrus): Astrigent used in diarrhoea.

मोहरी (Mohri) Mustard: It is useful against fevers due to Kuff. In small doses it liquifies the sputum. Externally it is counter irritant used as mustard poultice. In piles attended with itching and pain it allays these symptoms and reduces the size. Applied externally to the womb it contracts it.

Five (5) tolas are given in little water as emetic.

मंजिष्ट, (Manjist) मंजिष्ट, हिरडा, बेहडा, आवला, दारूहळद, Manjist, Hirda, Behda, Aowla, Daruhalad

बावर्डिंग, निशोत्तर, गुळेबल, कडूनिंब, zark, बेखंड,

Wawding, Nisator, Gulbe, Kadunimb, Bekhand.

Three (3) masas each or 45 grains each in 16 ounces of water, boil to 1/8th one ounce twice a day for 40 days. It is very useful to cure all kinds of skin diseases.

Mangist 2 tolas, sandal wood 2 tolas in 16 ounces of water boil to 1/8th one ounce twice a day given in urinary diseases. Promotes menstrual flow after parturition.

Externally it is used to relieve inflammation of sore eyes, and in acne erruptions on face and in burns.

यवक्षार, जवखार, (Yawakshar, Javakhar). It liquifies the sputum in 5 grain doses. It is also diuretic when taken as decoction in barley water. Mixed with त्रिफला, पुनर्नवा, धमासा, (Triphala, Punarnava, Dhamasa). It is useful in dropsy given as decoction in one ounce doses twice a day रक्तचंदन (Raktchandan) Red sandalwood. Externally it is applied in Erythema of skin धावरे (Dhawre) and to reduce inflammation in sore eyes. It is given in typhoid fevers रक्त चंदन, पदमकाष्ट, वाला, ध्ने, पित्तपापड़ा, नागरमोथा, गुलबेल, चिरायीत; Raktachandan, Patamkasht, Wala, Dhane, Pittpapda, Nagarmotha, Gulbel, Chirayeet, bark of कडूनिंब (Kadunimb) 10 grs. each in 16 ounces of water and boiled to 1/8th one ounce twice a day.

रक्तरोडा (Rakatroda): Extensively used in enlarged spleen.

रक्तरोडा (Rarkt roda) 2 tolas in 16 ounces of water, boil to 1/8th one ounce to be taken once a day.

रसांजन (Rasanjan). This is made after boiling from:

दारूहळद रसांजन (Daru, halad, rasanjan) grains 36 is made into small pills and taken with little milk. Stops Menorrhagia. It is used externally to reduce inflammation mixed with Alum and red sandalwood and to sore eyes. It is soluble in Rose water. Alum ½ tolas, ½ tolas catechu put in it 4 drops are put in the eyes twice a day.

रास्ना (Rasna)

रास्ना, गुलबेल, सोंठ, देवदार, एरंडमुल

Rasna, Gulbel, Sonth, Devdar, Arandmul.

Two tolas each in 16 ounces of water, boil to 1/8th, one ounce of this is mixed with castor oil 4 drs. taken early in the morning, useful in hemiplegia and all nervous diseases.

राल (Ral): It is astringent.

Grs. x Ral with little ghee and honey is given to stop diarrhoea in children. Externally it is used to keep broken ends of bones in apposition. It is boiled in little water and applied.

राल (Ral) one tola, मेण (Men) one tola, तिल्ली (Tilli) oil 2 tolas and boiled and then spread on a clean piece of cloth. It is also put in the fissures of the feet.

राल (Ral) one tola, पारा (Para) ¼ tola, coconut oil 7½ tolas, camphor ½ tola, केशर (Kesar) 1½ tolas, मोरचुत (Morchut) 15 grains boil and stir after adding water little by little and then draw off water and then put in मोरचूत (Morchut) 10 grs. draw off water and then mix with camphor and (Kesar) 5 grs. each. This ointment is used in all skin diseases.

रिठा (Ritha): Outer bark 15 grains is given to kill worms in children.

Inside of रिठा (Ritha) and ginger 1 gr. each is useful in Asthma.

रिठा, सागरगोटा (Ritha, Sagargota): Banduk seeds Asafoetidea ½ grain and black salt 1 gr. Ginger juice 10 drops, useful in stomach-ache. It is extensively used in epileptic fits. Ritha water is put in the nose or Ritha is burnt and put before the nose. It is also useful in hysteria. It is given as antidote against opium, aconite, arsenic and copper poisoning. It is rubbed in water and given and applied in snake and scorpion bites, externally. It is mixed with Asafoetida and applied externally in case of guinea-worms. It is mixed in water and put on the head and acts as ice bag.

रिंगणी (Ringni): It is against malarial fever.

रिंगणी, चिरायीत, सुंठ (Ringni, Chirayeet, Sonth) 1 dramch in 16 ounces of water one ounce is taken twice a day.

Ringni juice one tola and one tola ghee is given in dog bite poisoning.

रूई मदार (Rui, madar) Juice is cathartic purgative. Root one tola in 16 ounces of water boil to 1/8th, one ounce twice a day, useful against fevers with enlarged liver and cough.

नालगुंद (Nalgund): Take one rupee size of the leaf and mix 2 tolas of कुलीथ (Kulith) and 16 ounces of water, boil to 1/8th, 4 drs of this is given twice a day.

It is extensively used in Elephantiasis. Bark of the one tola, बेहड़ा (Behda) one tola, हिरडा (Hirda) one tola, आंवला (Anwla) one tola in 16 ounces of water boil to 1/8th, one ounce to be taken once a day for 40 days. Root is also well rubbed in butter milk and applied externally. Powdered root in 2 grs; doses is used as alternative in all sorts of skin diseases. Leaves are used externally in cases of distension of abdomen in children. Juice of madar is well rubbed in रेवाचिनी (Rewachini) and applied externally in case of enlarged glands.

रेणुक बीज (Renuk beej): It is a bazar medicine. It is very good against Hiccough. Powdered one tola is boiled in 16 ounces of water boil to 1/8th, one ounce twice a day useful in Hiccough.

Rewa chini given to children in one grain doses with little honey. It is aperient and emetic. Externally it is used on plague glands.

लवंग (Lavang) cloves.

They are stomachic, stimulant and appetiser. Extensively used in Asthma. Powdered cloves are useful in mucus diarrhoea. Pressed between the teeth it stops dental neuralgia.

लसुण (Lasun) Garlic: It is stimulant and useful in acid dyspepsia. Juice of लसुण (Lasun), ginger, and Asafoetida is useful in neuralgia. As a stimulant application in collapse with juice of betal and ginger juices. Juice in the ear stops ear-ache.

Garlic oil is useful in paralysis as external application. लाख (Lakh): It is good in whooping cough in 10 grs. doses. It also stops Hiccough with little honey. It is astringent and used in haemoptysis in 20 grs. doses twice a day. It is also used in tetany in children.

Oil is extracted as follows:

लाख (Lakh) 2 seers and 16 seers water, boil upto 4 seers, strain, add 4 seers of tilli oil and 16 seers of ताक (Tak) and mix हळद, देवदार, रास्ना, बडीशोप, जंष्टमध (Halad, Deodar, Rasna, Badisope, Jaishtmadh) 2 tolas each and boil slowly and stir and mix camphor 4 tolas. It is used in all cases of chronic fevers and in consumption.

लींबु (Limboo) Lemon: It is against Pitt.

Juice is prophylactic against cholera. It is used to reduce fat one tola of lemon juice in 10 tolas of hot water is taken after food for forty two days. It is extensively used in scurvy. In severe itching of the skin, juice one tola, is put in one ounce of coconut oil and well rubbed and then bathed with hot water it allays itching, used also in skin diseases. It is diuretic. Seeds are well rubbed in butter milk and applied over the umbilicus and then bathed with cold water useful in scanty micturition in children.

लोणी (Loni): Butter tonic one tola is given with little sugar. Butter one dr. and crystallised sugar one dramch is equal to one dr. of cod liver oil. Given with Pipeli one dr. and honey and sugar in consumption. Also given in piles. It allays the irritation.

Wawding वावडिंग grs. 10 in little water twice a day. It kills the worms and then after 2 doses it should be followed by castor oil as purgative, it is alterative Wawding 1 dr. Triphala one dr., Nishottar one dr., खडी साखर (Khari sakhar) one dr., to be taken every day in the morning acts as tonic alternative. It is also aperient.

It is a cooling medicine, powdered root grs. x with little milk and sugar allays burning sensation.

वाला, धने, बडीशोप (Bala, Dhane, Badishope) 30 grs. each, water 16 ounces boil to 1/8th and strain one ounce twice a day stops diarrhoea, promotes micturition and stops vomiting.

Vekhand वेखंडरू It is against worms, grs. x is taken in ताक (Tak). Stops colic, given with milk it promotes micturition, with Badishop it is aperient. It is extensively used in nervous diseases such as tetany, epilepsy etc. in proportionate doses. It is stimulant and ecbolic, बेखंड (Bekhand) 1 dr. with 10 grs. of sugar in little water promotes labour pains. Externally it is used mixed with camphor to promote healing of wounds and ulcers.

It is stimulant and stomachic and against cough. Decoction is used to stop vomiting with asafoetida, ginger and lemon juice is used in indigestion. Decoction with cloves is diuretic. It is extensively used in headache. 21 cardamoms and 2 drs. of Pipeli and then powdered to be taken in honey in headaches.

बेलु (Belu) Bamboo वंश लोचन (Vanshlochan).

30 grs. in little honey is given as a cooling medicine. Cinnamon one dr., cardamoms one dr., Pipeli one dr. and crystallised sugar one dr. is given in all kinds of fevers. It promotes micturition with Kanhal in equal proportion.

शतावरी (Shatawari) It is a diuretic. 4 tolas शतावरी (Shatawari) in 8 ounces of water boil to 1/8th, one ounce is given twice a day. Powdered one tola in milk stops leucorrhoea.

Oil of शतावरी (Shatawari): is used in epilepsy. Juice is extracted out of green herb and is mixed with tilli oil and 4 times cow's milk and boil. It is called Narayain oil of Shatawari. One tola of this oil is given in decoction of ginger in epilepsy and hysteria. It is used as cod liver oil in consumption and used in menstrual disorders. Juice from the roots one tola in 2 ounces of milk is a good diuretic and dissolves the stones. Decoction is made out of dry शतावरी (Shatawari).

शहाजिरा (Shahajira) given in diarrhoea in 20 grs doses. शिकाकाई (Shikakai): It is aperient and emetic. Shikakai one tola in 8 ounces of water decoction to 1/8th, one ounce twice a day. It is used against poisoning and in jaundice, externally it allays inflammation.

शेवगा (Shevga): It is stimulant. The bark reduces inflammation externally. Bark one tola water 8 ounces. Decoction to 1/8th and foment juice 4 drs mixed with Til oil 4 drs. is used to stop neuralgic pains and in headaches. Decoction of एरंड मुल शेवगा (Arand mool Shevga) one ounce each, water 16 ounces boil to 1/8th, one ounce twice a day useful in hemiplegia, white shevga seeds should be powdered and burnt and smoke inhaled. It stops headache.

शंखजिरा (Shankhjira): Astringent used in diarrhoea, used externally to promote healing of wounds.

सताप (Satap).

Juice 30 minims is given to children as tonic. It is against cough. It is used to promote menstrual flow in women. Juice is mixed with liquor and applied to the paralysed parts.

समुद्रफल (Samudraphal): It is a bazar medicine. It is an emetic. 2 or 3 drops are given in the teaspoonfull of juice of कारला अगस्ता (Karla Agasta) in children to promote vomiting.

साग (Sag): It reduces the inflammation externally and to reduce headache. Rubbed with little water and taken relieves indigestion. The seed is diuretic. It is stimulant to the hair applied to the head to promote hair growth.

Sagargota (Bonduck seeds)

It is extensively used in malarial fevers in 10 grs. doses and enlarged spleen. It kills worms when given with पलसपापड़ा (Palas papda) grs. x each in little honey. It is used to reduce inflammation externally rubbed in water. Inside of सागरगोटा (Sagargota) grs.x relieves stomach-ache given to women in puerperal state.

Sagargota one dr., Badishop one dr., white jira one dr., 20 grs of this to be taken early in the morning. Stops diarrhoea. Inside of Sagargota seeds grs. x Mire powdered one dr., Tulsi juice 1 dr. thrice a day, given in malarial fevers. It is also given with betal leaf in enlarged spleen.

सालम मिश्री (Salum misri): It is a tonic.

1/4 tola is given in 8 ounces of milk and two drs. of honey. It is also given with almonds and milk.

सुरन (Suran): It is good against piles. It is also stomachic सुरनपाक (Suranpak) is made of sugar and ghee.

सोरा (Sora) Potass nitras.

It should be dissolved in water and dried. Precipitate is again dried. It is diuretic and diaphoretic given in milk, it is used against cough. It is used externally dissolved in water to put on painful joints.

सोरा (Sora) 20 grs and 30 grs. Alum mixed in one tola ghee and sugar given twice a day stops leucorrhoea. It is extensively used in Asthma. Sora is dissolved in water and put on blotting paper and dried. The smoke is inhaled at the time of the fit. It is also mixed with the bark of Dhatura plant and cigarette made सोनामुखी (Sonamukhi).

It is a purgative, given in stomach-ache and worms (Thread worms). It is also diuretic. Decoction is given in dropsy and is used in piles. In small doses it is good against Asthma, Sonamukhi grs. xx, गोखरू (Gokhru) powders grs. xx, to be taken twice a day in little honey at bed time. It is a good aperient.

हळद (Halad): It purifies the blood. Halad 15 grs to be rubbed in 20 leaves of bitter Neem and taken only in the morning in little water for 7 days. It is also against worms in children. Halad 2 grs, wavding 2 grs, in little sugar to be given thrice a day against worms. Ten grs of Haldi with 10 grs of til with little sugar stops excessive micturition, 10 grs of haldi mixed with curd is useful in Jaundice, mixed in milk in 5 gr. in 8 ounces it is useful against cough, and in cow's ghee it is against poisoning. Externally, reduces the inflammation. 5 tolas of Halad in 8 ounces of water boil and put on the sore eyes. It is also applied over the piles rubbed in water, catechu and Halad in small-pox externally. Halad is disinfectant. It is also tonic in 5 grs. doses taken in little milk at night.

हस्तिदंत (Hastidant): Ivory ashes are mixed in रसांजन (Rasanjan) and applied to the head to produce hair.

Ferrisulph. हिराकस (Hirakas) green coloured one is used in medicine. It is fried in ghee and kept in bottle. Hirakas grs 2, Pipeli grs 2 and honey one dr. used as tonic, acid things are to be avoided. If there be constipation little castor oil is given as aperient.

Ferrisulph grs. 3 and Triphala 30 grs. is given in anaemia. Ferrisulph grs. 3, Inf. Chiretta one dr., Pipeli grs. V is useful in enlarged spleen. Given, in decoction of त्रिफला (Triphala) 1/8th in 3 grs., doses, one ounce twice a day useful in bleeding piles.

हिरडा (Hirda) grs. x in little honey is tonic. It is given in sugar, ginger or honey.

Decoction of 6 Hirda in 16 ounces of water boil to 1/8th. To be taken early in the morning. It produces 3 or 4 motions in case of piles and in muscus diarrhoea. It is also given in breathlessness and cough in 10 gr, doses in little honey. Decoction one ounce is given in headache and in eye affections it is given in grs. x doses mixed with honey and ghee.

Ayurvedic Drugs for Following Diseases

Indigestion: Butter milk, pudina, Ammo, chloride, badishop, garlic.

Diarrhoea: Isabgol, camphor, poppy seeds, mayphal, Sagargota, Banduck seeds.

Acidity: Ginger, Anwla, Lime water, grapes, Hirda.

Opium Poisoning: Dewdala.

Tastelessness: Anwla, kokumb, mirchi.

Half headache: Anwla, vekhand.

Debility: Urad grain, musk, butter, salum misri, hirakas hirda.

अगरू (*Ageru*): Alum and marking nut.

Tetany of Children: Camphor, gorochan, cloves, vekhand, akkalkhada.

Acid Dyspepsia आम्लवात *(Amlawat)*—Camphar, lime water black salt, badishop, hirda, guggul.

Mucoid Dyspepsia आमांश *(Amansh)*—Castor oil, onion, jambul, daru halad, mayphal, ral, isabgol.

Loss of Voice—Jestha madh, catechu, betal leaves.

Eczema—Dambar and coconut.

Hiccough आकी, अहारन *(Aki, Aharan)*—Ahaliv tulas dhamasa, garlic.

Boil and Ulcers—Umber, onion, palas and shewga.

Rat Bite Poisoning—Marking nut, aghada.

Dropsy—Castor oil, पुनर्नवा (punarnava), यवक्षार (yawkshar), senna.

Delirium—Ammo. chloride, नवसागर (navsagar), ritha, betal leaves.

Scanty mecturition उन्हाळे *(Unhale)*—Aghada, मेहंदी, गोखरू (mehndi, gokhura), sandalwood, kankol, grapes.

Syphilis उपदंश *(Updansh)*—Bark of neem tree, कांचन ब्राम्ही (kanchan, brahmi), upal-sari.

Haemoptysis उरःक्षत *(Urahshat)*—Ammo. chloride, जेष्टमा (Jaishtmadh), grapes, gopichandan.

Vomiting—Ginger, dikemali, lime water, tamarind, jeshtmadha, badishop, lemon juice.

Emetic—गेलफल, बेखंड (gelphal, Bekhand).

Heated Sensation in the Body—Figs, butter, grapes, lotus, bakul palas, mehndi.

Itching sensation—करंज (Karanj) and cocum oil, halad, ambehalad, sulphar.

Cough—Jambul, jeshthmadha, hirda, alum, ammo. chloride, palas, maka.

Lumago—Akkalkhara, mustard, rewachini, marking nut, ahaliv and satap.

Chicken-pox—Behada, jeshthmadha and grapes.

Ear-ache—Juice ginger, garlic and takankhar.

Jaundice—Daruhalad, ammo. chloride, biroja, मेंदी, मंजीष्ट, शीकाकाई (mendi, manjisht and shikakai).

Cholera—Onion, tamarind, jambul, mirchi, jayaphal and lemon.

Dogbite poisoning—Aghada, lime, ringni, betel-leaves.

Hair Restorer—Jaswand, til, jatamasi and kachora.

Leucoderma—Kadubewachi, Papai, outer covering of Coconut, Nishottar, Chitrak, Bark of Neem tree.

Skin disease कुष्ट *(Kusht)*—Karanj, Blue-Lotus, Marking Nut, Madar and Wavding.

Scabies—Oil of Karanj and Neem, Sulphur, Lime, Sandal wood oil, Ral, Halad, and Bawachi.

Granulations—Alum, Palas, Papdi, Tarwad.

Cough—Kakadshingi, Kankol.

Whooping Cough—Taknkhar, Pipeli, Ammo.-chloride, Nagarmotha, Yawakhar, Ringni, Aghada. Betal-leaves,

Abortion—Jaswand.

Boils on the Body—Camphor, Guggul, Lineseed,

Enlarged Glands—Karaj, Apta, Gandhabiroja.

Mumps—Umber, Lime, Lemon, Guggul, Ammo.-chloride.

Dyspepsia—Ginger, Pipeli, Bangaddhar, Salt Senna.

Measles—Camphor, Gorochan, Mendi. Potass. nitre.

*Burning in the Throa*t—गोपीचन्दन (Gopichandan), and Geru.

Diseases of throat—कंकोल (Kankol) and cloves.

Profuse perspiration—Aniseed, Ginger, Mosk and pipeli.

Diaphoretics—Camphor, Tulas, Dewdar, Dhana, Kulith.

Chai—Jaswand.

Wounds—Lineseed, Wax, Mendi, Catechu, Shankhjira, Ambehalad.

Worms—Indrajava, Gelphal, Dikemali, Papai, Palas, Wawding, Vekhand, Ritha, Kirmani owa.

Dropsy—Juice from Plantain tree and Hirda.

Neuralgia—Cocum oil, Gokkaru, Alum, Mendi, Ral,

Insomnia—Dhamasa, Mendi, Onion, Jayaphal,

Baldness—Jaswand, Maka, Ashes of Ivory, Gandhabiroja.

Loss of Appetite—Juice of Karla.

Headache—Camphor, Takankhar, Grapes, Tulas, Ammon. chloride, Vekhand, Hirda, Sag.

Diseases of the Eyes—Camphor, Alum, Daruhalad, Makka, Rasanjan, Raktachandan, Lemon.

Dengu Fever—निरगुंडी (Nirgundi).

Thirst—Cloves, Sora, Jeshthmadh, Dhane, Nagarmotha, Coconut water, Grapes.

Influenza—Indrajaba, Kakadshinghi, Camphor, Gulbel, Sandalwood, Takankhar, Ammo. chloride, Bharangmul, Shevga, Bundack seeds, सागरगोटा (Sagargota), निशोत्तर (Nishottar).

Mouth Diseases—Jambul, Alum, Pudina, Rasanjan, Jeshtmadh, Manjistha.

Ulcers in the Mouth—Alum, Kaw, Jeshthmadh.

Paralysis of Face—Udid, Camphor.

Asthma—Aghada, Takankhar, Pipeli, Ammo. chloride, Garlic, Potass. nitrate, Ritha, Camphor, Kankol, Dhamasa.

Dental Caries—Takankhar, Bakul, Mayaphal, Ringni, Mire, Cloves, Akkalkadha, Khair.

Burning Sensation in the Body—Dhane, Coconut, Vala, Sandalwood, Grapes, Badishope.

Alcoholic Intoxication—Decoction of Grapes.

Small-pox—Camphor, Neem leaves, Rose, Gorochan, Mendi, Adulsa, Catechu.

धावरे *(Dhaware)* or *Erysipelas*—Kaw Kanchan, Bakul, Red Sandalwood.

Leucorrhoea—Camphor, Malkangani, Shatawari, Isabgul, Jaswand, Daruhalad, Alum, Ral, Rasanjan, Awala, Bole, Ritha.

Phosphoturia—Gokharu, Mosk, Chopchini and Grapes.

Urticaria—Neem leaves, Sulphur, Ral, Lakh, Wavding, Takla, Lemon juice.

Guinea-worm—Askanth, Lime, Ritha.

नालगुंद एरंड *(Nalgund Arand)*—Root of castor oil plant, Kulith and Madar.

Cold—Akkalkadha, Tulas, Halad, Cinnamon, Dewdar.

Gonorrhoea—Camphor, Kankol, Sandalwood, Jahu, Ral, Biroza, Nim bark.

Anaemia पांडूरोग *(Pandurog)*—Butter-milk, Grapes, Ammo. chloride, Nishottar.

Diseases of the Nose—Guggul, Jai, Mustard, Kosht.

For Excess of Bile पित्त *(Pitt)*—Isabgol, Sugar cane, Lotus, Kokumb, Tamarind, Pomogranate, Dhane, Mendi, Rasanjan, Lemons.

For Skin Diseases पैठ *(Paitha) dry Eczema.* Oil of Karanj.

Stomach—Jambul, Bol, Murudsheng, Ritha, Vekhand, Indrajava, Pipeli, Takankhar, Lemon,

Distension of Stomach—Pipeli, Badishop, Bangadkhat, Bol, Garlic, Senna, Hirda, Ginger.

For Urinary Diseases—Sandalwood, Owa, Jambul, Til, Alum.

To Dissolve Hair in the Stomach—Juice of अननस (Ananas.)

Enlarged Spleen—Ammo. chloride, Pipeli, Ferri-sulph Ambehalad, Bunduck Seeds, सागरगोटा (Sagargota), Aghada, Hirda.

Plague—Camphor, Chittrak, Mustard.

Epilepsy, Hysteria—Musk, Onion, Camphor, Kosht, Bramhi, Cloves, Vekhand, Shatawari, Shewga, Akkalkadha.

Fistula भगंदर *(Bhahgander)*—Karanj oil, Badishop, Korphad.

Burns—Lime water, Catechu, Lineseed, or Tilli oil, Sandalwood, Korphad.

Giddiness— Awala, Grapes, Dhamasa, Ginger, Coconut.

Bhowari भोवरी *(Bhonwri)*-Dhamasa.

Diabetes मधुमेह *(Madhumeh)*—Kanchan, Jambul, Takala Butter-milk, Marking nut.

Constipation, मलावरोध (Malavroadh)—Figs, Castor oil Sulphur, Tamarind, Nishottar, Hirda, Isabgul.

Leprosy—Kadu, Bawacha.

Watering in the Mouth—Jambul, Tarwad.

मुर्मे *(Murme)*—Jambul.

Fainting मुच्छीं *(Murchchi)*—Musk, Onion, Ritha, Brahmi, Ritha Salt.

Stoppage of Micturition—Apta, Cane juice, Gokharu, Dhamasa, Bakul, Butter-milk, Grapes, Till, Aghada, Pot. nitre., Shatawari.

Alkaline Urine—Lineseed, Gokharu, Punarnava, Kankol, Vekhand, Nagarmotha, Biroza.

Piles—Onion, Guggul, Sulphur, Daruhalad, Biroza, Bahawa, Mayaphal, Alum, Malkangani, Halad, Nagkeshar, Ferrisulph, Hirda.

Copper Sulphate, Poisoning—Lemon (Citrous juice. Obesity. Kalingad, Karanj, Guggul, honey, Hirda, Maka, Lemon, and Catechu.

Englarged liver Dropsy—Ammo., chloride, Korphal, Pipeli, and Chittruk.

Rakat Pitt—Grapes, Upalsari, Gopichandan, Jeshtamadh, Bahawa.

To Reduce Inflammation—Ambehalad, Korphad.

Blood Purifier—Bark of Neem, Upalsary, Jatamansi, Korphad.

Scorpion Bite—Agadha, Apta, Alum and Betal leaves.

Amenorrhoea—Keshar, Koshta Ammo. chloride, Papai.

Antidote to Poisoning—Gelphal, Takankhar, Tulus, Dewdali, Ritha, Vekhand, Shikakai, Halad.

Englarged Scrotum—Karanj, Nirgundi, Gandh-Biroza, Sagargota.

Insanity—Khursani Owa.

Fistula—Takankhar Biroza, Maka, Ral, Haladi, Catechu.

Tenaea Versicolour—Kadu Bawcha, Kadu Kawathi.

Contraction of Muscles—Til and Garlic oil.

Neuralgia—Camphor, Marking nut, Guggul, Ginger, Juice.

Diarrhoea संग्रहणी (Sangrahni)—Kakadshingi, Poppy seeds, Chittrak, Takankhar, Ammonium chloride, Grapes, Kaw.

Snake Poisoning—Dewdali, Betal leaves.

Internal Inflammation—Punarnawa, Bakul, Bahawa, Rasanjan, Shevga, Sag, Ferri. Sulph., Ambehalad, Biroza.

Arsenical Poisoning.—Isabgol.

Night Emissions—Camphor, Chopchini, gokhru.

Intoxication from Betalnut—Kalingad.

Fractures—Guggul, Red sandalwood, Arjunsadad.

Heart Disease—Lotus, Bel, Garlic, Camphor, Honey, Agastha, Pomogranate and Dhane.

Consumption—Lotus, Adulsa, Grapes, Pipeli, Bamboo leaves, Kolphad, Gulbel.

Astringent Drugs—Allum, Asokebark, Babul gum, Bael, Butea gum, Catechu, Kurchi bark, Myrobolans, Beheda-Myrobolans (Embelic) Awla, opium, Bark of pomogranate.

Antiscorbutice—Papai, Tamarind.

Antispasmodics—Asafoetida, Borax (Sohag), Dhatura, Opium.

Carminatives—Aniseed, Cinnamon, Cloves, Ginger, Nutmeg, Pipal, Turmeric.

Demulsions—Gokhru, Isabgol, Kakadsinghi Liquorice.

Diuretics—Kababchini (cuoebs), Galancha, Pot. nitras.

Emetic—Mudar, Mustard, Salt, Copper Salphate.

Expectorants—Ammo. chloride, Kakadshinghi, Mudar, Myrrh.

Purgatives—Alubokhara, Castor oil, Kaladana, Senna, Sulphur.

Sedatives—Asafoetida, Borax (Sohaga), Dhatura, Opium.

Tonics—Bunduck-seeds (Sagar-gota), Chalmogra oil, Atia Gokharu, Nembbark, Sulphate of Iron.

Alternatives: Chiretta, Chobchini, Indian Sarsa parila.

Anthelmintic: Butea seeds, Papai fruit, Promogranate root bark.

Some Ayurvedic Prescription

Hysteria:	Camphor	grs. 2.
	Aloes	grs. 2.
	Asafoetida	grs. 2
	Jatamansi	grs. 5.

Honey 1 dr. To be taken twice a day.

Influenza:	Long pepper (Pipul)	grs. 2.
	Asefoetida	gr. 1.
	Kakodshinghi	gr. 1.
	Liquorice	gr. 1.
	Gum	gr. 1.

Make one pill, to be taken three times a day.

Laxative Powder, Powdered Senna leaves grs. 10.

Myrobolan (Har)	grs. 10.
Liquorice	grs. 20.
Caraway Jira	grs. 10.

To be taken at bed time with little water.

Malarial Fever: Bunduck seed powder	grs. 10.
Kaladana	grs. 10.
Black pepper	grs. 5.

Fiat powder. One powder to be taken twice a day with little honey,

Powder for Piles: Myrobolans (har)   grs. 20.
          Bellaric (Behada) Myrobalans   grs. 15.
          Embelic Myrobalans Awala   grs. 15.
          Kaldana   grs. 5.
          Senna leaves   grs. 15.

Fiat, powder, to be taken at bed time in 8 ounces with hot water.

Purgative: Myrobalans (Choti Har)   drs. 2.
              Cinnamon   dr. 1.
              Kaladana   grs. 20.
              Rhubarb (Rewachini)   dr. 1.

To be taken early in the morning, in 2 drs. of honey or water.

For Rheumatic Joints: Lemon grass. oil   1 oz.

Juice of Ginger 1 drs. Camphor 2 drs, Sweet oil 4 ozs.

Joint to be well rubbed twice a day

Enlarged Spleen: Rewachini Rhubarb.   5 grs.
                 Hirakas   2 grs.
          Embelic Myrobalans (Har)   10 grs.

To be taken at bed time.

Tape worm: Root bark of Promogranate fresh   2 ozs.
             Water.   40 ozs.

Boil to 1/2. Dose 2 ozs. in the morning, fasting, repeat every half hour for four days, then a dose of Castor oil.

Tonic. Ferri Sulph — 2 grs.
    Ind. Sarsaparilla (Anantmul) Decoction — 1 oz.
Boiled 10 ozs. of water to half.
    To be taken twice a day.
Bitter Tonic: Decoction of Neem bark — 4 ozs.
    Decoction of Cloves — 1 oz.
    Infusion Chiretta — 3 drs.
One ounce to be taken twice a day.
Uterine Haemorrhage. Decoction of Asoke Bark 4 ozs
    boiled in water 20 ozs. to 1/4 — 4 ozs
    Alum — 5 grs.
Decoction of Babool bark 4 drs. thrice a day.

Ayurvedic Prescriptions

1. For Itch: Babool leaves six ounces burnt and mixed with Kerosene oil and applied to the skin.

2. Frequent Micturition: आष्टा (Ashta) seeds one tola or 3 drachms soaked in water and drunk with little sugar.

3. To Hasten Suppuration: Inside of Sitaphal सीताफल 2 oz, Rock salt 4 drs. to be applied externally over the boils.

4. For Guinae worm: Pounded leaves of सीताफल (Seetaphal) to be applied over it.

5. Dyspepsia. Powdered Galic — grs. x
    " Jira — grs x.
    " Padelon — grs x.
    " Ginger — grs. x.
    " Pipeli — grs. x.

	Fried Asafoetida	
	Lemon juice	drs. 2.

To be taken early in the morning.

6. *Choleric Diarrhoea:*

Garlic	grs. 5
Jira	grs. 5
Ginger	grs. 5
Fried Asafoetida	grs. 5
Opium	gr. 1/2
Mirchi	grs. 2
Honey	dr. 1

fiat powder to be taken every 3rd hour.

7. *Diabetes:* Jambul seeds powdered 1 dr, milk 1 ounce to be taken twice a day.

8. *Mouth Wash:* Inner bark of Jambul, Babul, Bukul and Bel one ounce each, water 16 ounces, boil to 1/8th, and teeth to be rubbed with powdered bark of Bakul.

9. *Chronic Diarrhoea:* Juice of Jambul 1 dr. to be taken in little water thrice a day.

10. *Diabetes:*

Powder Jambul seeds	1 drs.
Black Til	2 drs.
Chopchini	1 dr.
Gokhru	1 dr.
Khus-khus	1 dr.
Hirda	1 dr.
Behada	1 dr.
Awla-kathi	1 dr.
Amber	15 grs.
Honey	2 drs.

To be taken twice a day.

11. Menorrhagia: One once decoction of inner bark of Jambul tree twice a day, Jambul bark one ounce, water 16 oz, boil to 1/8th.

12. Hiccough: Jambul juice one drachm. Akkal-kadha, grs 5, Pimpali grs. 4.

13. Diarrhoea with Blood: Juice of Jambul, Mango and Awla leaves 1 drachm, to be taken in little honey and milk.

14. Leprosy: अनंतमूल (Anantmul) 1 drachm, to be rubbed in little water and taken in the morning.

बेल पाडल मूल (Welpadalmul) 1 drachm, to be rubbed in cold water and taken in the noon.

सर्प संधी मूल (Sarpsandhimul) 1 drachm, to be rubbed in cold water and taken in the evening.

15. Scanty Micturition: Ashes of Tilli plant grs 10 to be taken with little water twice a day.

16. Polyuria. Abundance of urine.

Powdered Jambul seeds grs x, thrice a day with little water.

17. Jaundice: Juice of castor oil plant 1 dr, milk one ounce twice a day.

18. Dental Pain. Camphor grs 10, Allum grs 10, pot. nitrate grs. 10, Ammonium chloride (Nawasagar) grs 10 and Hirda grs. 10 to be rubbed over this morning and, evening.

19. Cholera: 2 drops of marking nut oil, milk one ounce to be given every two hours.

20. Dry Eczema: Rock salt grs, xx Kadu nimb leaves 2 ounces.

This is to be applied externally to soften it and then the following ointment, white catechu. 4 drachms, Ral 4 drs., Siras oil one ounce, wax 4 drs. to be applied externally.

21. Balghuti: Powder... grs 3, Beheda grs. 3, Indrajava one grain, Wawding... Akkalkadha grs 2, Jeshtamadh grain one, Rock salt g... one. To be given in little water twice a day.

22. Mouth wash for ulceration in the mouth: Babul bark 4 ounces, water 15 ounces boil to 1/8th and strain to 1/8th and put 30 grs of Alum. To be taken twice a day.

बालंतकाढा (Balantkadha): Tonic for women in Puerperal state.

Dewadar, Vekhand, Sunth, Kayphal, Nagarmotha, Chiretta, Katuki, Dhane, Shingani, Gokhru, Dhamasa, Gulbel Inside of bail fruit, Shahjira one tola each, make 14 powders, and add 16 ozs of water and boil to 8th and strain and put in one drachm of ghee, 60 grains of rock salt and 10 grains Asafoetida. One oz. of this to be taken twice a day.

Acidity: Gulvel 1 oz., bitter, Padwal 1 oz., Pittpapada 1 dr., Adulsa 1 oz., add 16 ozs. of water and boil to 1/6th. Half an ounce to be taken twice a day.

Leucorrhoea: Five flowers of Gulkhairi गुलखैरी (gulkhairi) to be pounded with sugar and taken once in the morning.

Bleeding Piles: External application of seeds of मालकंगनी (Malkaugani).

Granulations in the Eyes: काडीखार (Kadikhar) grs. 10 to be dissolved in rose water 1 oz. and put in the eyes.

Enlarged-Spleen: Juice of कोरफड़ (Korphad) 1 dr. mixed in little Haldi taken in morning and evening.

डबा (Daba, powdered वृन्दावन Wrandawan grs. 2 and, honey 1 dramch, twice a day.

Tetanus: Cloves 15, Jayphal one tola, Ginger 3 toals, root of Jangali Tulas one tola, made in 7 pills. One pill once in the morning.

Syphilis: Dhayati flowers one tola, Khurasani owa one tola, Kirmani owa one tola, Marking nut one tola, Cloves one tola, Jayapatri one tola, Jayphal one tola, Mercury grs. 10 to be rubbed in Sasafron grs. 10, make 30 pills as such, one pill to be taken twice a day in little curd.

Malarial-fever:		
Bark of Kuda tree...		1 oz.
Takala root	...	1 oz.
Adulsa	...	1 oz.
Gulbel	...	2 oz.
Ringni	...	1 oz.
Water	...	60 oz.

Boil to 1/2 (half), 1/2 an ounce to be taken twice a day Or:—

Hingul	...	gr.	1/20.
Arsenic	...	gr.	1/100.
Catechu	...	grs.	5.
Betal nut juice	...		1 dr.

To be taken once a day.

Tuberculosis:			
	Camphor	...	grs. 5
	Saffron	...	grs. 2
	Khuskhus	...	grs. 5

Mulethi	...	grs. 5
Seeds of turbuz.	...	grs. 5

Powder. One powder to be taken in little honey twice a day.

Asthma:

Madar-kikali	...	gr. 1
Pipal	...	gr. 1
Rock salt	...	gr. 1

Fiat. Pill one pill twice a day.

Dysentery:

Mucilage-Ispghul	...	1 dr.
Mucilage-Bhinhi	...	1 dr.
Aqua-add	...	1 oz.

one ounce twice a day.

Corneal Opacity & Plerygium.

Red Sandalwood	...	2 dr.
Beheda.	...	2 drs.
Palas gum.	...	3 drs.

Powder and mix to be applied twice.

Rheumatism:

Badam mugz.	...	2 drs.
Leaves of mehndi	...	2 drs.
Sasafron	...	1 dr.
Sugar	...	4 drs.

Dose 30 grains twice a day.

Scurvy

Dried Amchur	...	1 dr.
Tamarind	...	1 dr.

To be taken twice a day.

Diseases of Respiratory System

Bronchitis. Powdered   Pepper   ... 1 dr.
              "   Kakadsingi.   1 dr.
              "   Cloves   ... 1 dr.
              "   Pipal   ... 1 dr.
              "   Ginger   ... 1 dr.
              "   Rock salt   1 dr.

Make 20 pills, one pill three times a day.

Dyspnoea: Camphor   ... grs. 2.
              Ginger   ... grs. x.
              Khaskhas safed ... grs. x.
              Honey   ... 1 dr.

To be taken twice a day.

Emphysema: Powdered Jawkbar. ... grs. 10
   Ammonium chloride (nawasagar)   grs. 5
   Honey   ... 1 ds.

Twice a day.

Laryngitis: Powdered Khurasani Ajawan. grs. 10
           "   Pipal   ... grs. 10
           "   Malkangani   ... grs. 10

Twice a day.

Tuburcle of Lung.

              Wasantmalti ... gr. 1
              Honey   ... 1 dr.

Thrice daily.

Diseases of Digestive System

Dyspepsia.	Powdered Pepper	...	grs. 10
"	Pipal	...	grs. 10
"	Anardana	...	grs. 10
"	Jawakhar	...	grs. 10
"	Sugar	...	1 dr.

To be taken twice a day.

Jaundice: Kasundi leaves 1 gr., Kali mirch 1 dr. pound and mix some water, twice daily.

Spogy-gums: Alum grs. 10, Akarkadha grs. 10, Pepper grs.10, Honey 4 drs. mix, to be applied to gums.

Vomiting: Camphor	...	...	grs. 5
Kurchi	...	...	grs. 2

Worms: Bark of Papai 1 oz., water 16 osx., boil to 1/8th, one ounce to be taken at bed time on an empty stomach, useful in thread and Tape worms.

Diseases of Genito-urinary-System

For urethral irritation. Alum grs. 10, Copper sulphate grs. 3 and water add one ounce.

Gonorrhoea: Safed Wansh-jochan	...	grs. 5
Kusta katar (Oxide of Tin)	...	gr. 1
Kabab-chini (Cubebs)	...	grs. 5
Safed Elaichi (Cardamom)	...	grs. 10
Honey	...	1 dr.

To be taken twice a day.

Impotence: Salum-mishri ... grs. 5

Talmakhana	...	grs. 2
Indrajava	...	grs. 2
Cinnamom	...	grs. 2
Almonds	...	grs. 30
Honey	...	2 drs.

Twice a day.

Renal and vescicle calculus.

Gokharu powdered	...	1 dr.
Linseed seeds	...	1 dr.
Sugar	...	2 drs.

Twice a day.

Diseases of Nervous System

Apoplexy: Juice of the root of Chukunder, a few drops to be put in the nose.

Epilepsy:	Akar kadha	...	grs. 10
	Guggul	...	grs. 5
	Pepper	...	grs 10
	Sunflower seeds	...	gr. 1
	Honey	...	1 ds.

Twice a day.

During an epileptic fit put in few drops of juice of bitter Turai (Kadu-Dodaka) in the nose.

Hemiplegia and Facial Paralysis.

Akarkhara	...	grs. 5
Pepper	...	grs. 5
Pimpalmul	...	grs. 2
Ginger	...	grs. 5

Pound and mix with butter and gur to be takan twice a day.

Insomnia: Khaskhas. ... 1 dr.
Badam ... grs. 30
Sugar ... 1 ds.

To be taken 3 or 4 times a day.

Vertigo: Khaskhas safed ... 1 ds
Champhor ... grs. 2
Dhania ... grs. 5
Honey ... grs. 2

Twice a day.

Diseases of Skin

Alopecia. Mustard oil ... 2 drs.
Awla oil ... 2 drs.
Almond oil ... 2 drs.
Mehndi oil ... 2 drs.
Decotion Lal mirch ... 1 dr.

The part to be well rubbed twice a day.

Bed sores: Mustard oil ... 2 drs.
Saindur ... 30 grs.
Mehndi leaves ... 2 drs.

Make a paste and apply.

Dhobis itch: Sulphur ... 1 dr.
Saindur ... grs. 20
Safeda ... grs. 20
Haldi ... 1 dr.

Mix with butter and apply:

Eczema:

Ral	...	2 drs.
Wax	...	2 drs.
Hartal	...	1 dr.
Mustard oil	...	2 ounces

Apply on the affected parts twice a day after washing it with carbolic soap and hot water.

Leprosy:

Mercury (Para)	...	gr. 1/2
Arsenic (Sankhia)	...	1/100
Rewa chini	...	grs. 10
Babul gum	...	dr. 1
Lemon juice	...	dr. 1

To be taken twice a day.

Leucoderma:

Allum	...	1 dr.
Sora	...	1 dr.
Hirakas	...	1 dr.
Venegar	...	2 ozs.

Apply twice a day.

Babchi. Pound and make a paste with water and apply. The blood of a black snake is the best local application over the patches of leucoderma.

Pesoriasis Versicolour (Shibe)

Champa flowers and juice of lemon.

For external application.

Ring-worm:

Hartal.	...	1 dr.
Sulphur	...	1 dr.
Sweet oil	...	1 dr.

Make an ointment for external application.

Scabies. Sulphur ... 2 drs.
  Safeda ... 1 dr.
  Cow's milk. ... 2 ozs.
  Ghee ... 1 oz.

Put on fire and make into an ointment.

Urticaria: Chironj ... 2 drs. to be well rubbed in
  Cocum oil ... 1 oz.

To be rubbed over the body.

Diseases of the Ear

Ear-ache: Juice of the leaves of Raddish muli. 1 dr.
  Sweet oil. 1 dr.

One or two drops to be put in the ears.

Deafness: Juice of onion 2 drops warm to be put in the ear.

Inflammation of Tympanic Membrane

  Mustard Oil ... ms. v.
  Camphor ... grs. 2.
  Brandy ... ms, xx.

2 or 3 drops to be put in the ear after fomenting.

Diseases of the Eye

Cataract. Blister to be temple.

Ammo: chloride. (Navsagar) grs. 10 powdered and mixed with honey one ounce for local application to the eye.

Corneal opacity: Red sandalwood ... grs. 10
  Rock salt ... grs. 10

Beheda	...	grs. 10
Gum of Palas	...	grs. 40

Powder and mix.

Night blindness. Juice of leaves of Saras 2 or 3 drops to be put in the eyes mixed with little water.

Diseases of the Women

Abortion: (Preventive) Decoction of babool bark one ounce in 16 ounces of water 4 drs. to be taken twice a day.

Amenorrhoea: (Kapas (cotton) root ... 1 ounce.
               Water 16 ounces boil to ... 1/8 th

One ounce to be taken twice a day.

Hysteria: Asafoetida ... grs. 3
         Camphor ... grs. 3
         Musk ... gr. 1
         Honey ... dr. 1

Twice a day.

Leucorrhoea: Salum misri ... grs. 20
            Powdered Khaskhas ... grs. 20
            Powdered Badam ... 2 drs.
            Decoction Jaswand root bark ... 1 dr.
            Sugar ... 2 drs.
            Goat's milk ... 1 ounces

To be taken twice a day.

Menorrhagia: Root of Gular one ounce.
             Water two seers.
             Boil to 1/8th one ounce to be taken twice a day

Fistula in Ano: Safed Mom. ... 4 drs.
Opium ... grs. 4
Murdad-sheng powdered. ... 1 dr.

For local application.

Prolapse: Decoction of babool bark and betal leaves in equal parts.

For external application.

Forround-worm Asafoetida ... grs. 1
Chiretta powder ... grs. V
Butea seeds powdered ... grs. 5

To be taken at bed time.

Vomiting of cholera: Lemon grass oil ... ms. 3
Camphor ... gr. 1.

In half teaspoonfull of sugar thrice a day.

Ring-worm: Sohaga (Boracis) one ... dr. 1
Sulphate of copper. ... grs. V
Linseed oil ... 4 drs.

To be applied over the affected part twice a day.

Stomach colic: Asafoetida ... grs. 1
Black pepper ... gr. 1
Ajwain seeds powdered ... gr. 1
Cardamom ... gr. 1
Mucilage acasia. ... q. s.

Misce flat pill to be taken twice a day.

Acidity: Slaked lime (Chuna) 1/2 ounce.
Water two points.

Shake well and allow to deposit for 12 hours. Mix with equal parts of milk. One ounce to be taken twice a day.

Cholera pill:

	Ginger	...	grs. 3
	Red pepper	...	gr. 1
	Asafoetida	...	gr. 1
	camphor	...	gr. 1
	Opium	...	gr. 1/2

Make one pill to be taken thrice a day.

Diaphoretic and Antiperiodic

Barberry root (Rasaut)	4	ounces
Chiretta (Chirait)	4	"
Ajwon (Carum)	60	grains
Pot Nitrate (Sora)	160	"
Water	40	ounces
Boil to 1/2		

One ounce to be taken twice or thrice a day.

Diarrhoea and Dysentery

Pomogranate Rind of fruit (Bruised) (Anar)	2 ounces
Water	20 Drachm

Boil for 15 minutes and add Catechu (Katho) 10 grains, Cinnomon (Dalchini) 10 grains, Butea Gum (Palas) 5 grains.

One ounce to be taken twice a day.

Astringent Mixture for Diarrhoea

Catechu Katho bruised	1 drachms
Cinnamon (Dalchini) bruised	1 drachms
Macerate for two hours and	5 grs.

strain, add allum.

One source to be taken twice a day.

Digestive

Choti har	...	20 grains
Behera	...	20 "
Auwla	...	20 "
Asafetida	...	1 grain.
Caraway (Jira)	...	3 grains
Carum (Ajwan)	...	3 "
Lahori Salt (Sendha Nimak)		3 "

Misce.

One powder to be taken at bed time.

Digestive Powder

Soda Bicarb	...	10 grains
Rhubarb (Rewa Chini)	...	5 "
Ginger	...	5 "

To be taken at bed time.

Dropsy

Potassium Nitrate (Shora)	10 grains
Infusion Moringa root (Shajna)	1 ounce
Barbria root (Asteracantha)	4 drachms
Water ...	20 Ounce.

Boil for 10 minutes and strain, one ounce twice a day.

Dusting Powder

Boracic Acid (Sohaga).	1 drachm.

Sank jira powdered	...	1 ”
Starch	...	1 ”
Oxide of Zinc	...	1 ”

Dysentry

Isabgolul finely powdered	30 grains
Anisiseed ”	30 ”
Boil ”	30 ”
Liquorice (Mulathi) ...	10 grains
Fennel fruit (Bari Sonf)	10 ”

To be taken twice a day.

Emetic

Copper Sulphate (Tutya)	4 grains
Water ...	4 drachms

One teaspoonfull every 10 minutes, for four doses.

Flatulent Colic

Dalchini	10 grains
Elachi	10 ”
Asafoetida	1 gr.

To be taken twice a day.

Gonorrhoea

Shora (Potassium nitrate)	10 grs.
Decoction of fresh (Bhindi)	2 ounces.

One ounce to be taken twice a day.

Headache

Camphor	...	1 ounce

Vinegar (Sirka)	...	8 ounces

To be applied externally.

Vinegar	...	1 ounce
Water	...	4 ounces

For sponging the body in fevers.

For Anaemia

Sulphate of Iron (Kasis)		2 grains
Black Pepper (Kala Mirach)		2 grains
Aloes (Mussabar)	...	1 grain
Asafoetida	...	1 "
Gum Accacis	...	q. s.

One pill to be taken twice a day.

Apthae

Borax	...	1 dr.
Honey	...	1 ounce

Apply with cotton wool to the mouth.

Bed Sores

Boracis (Sohaga)	...	1 dr.
Wax (Mom)	...	1 ounce
Piney Resin (Sufed damur)	...	4 "
Fat	...	4 "

Heat gently and stir while cooling.

For Blister

Root Bark (Lalchitra) fresh		2 drs.
Flour of rice and water sufficient for a paste, apply on a cloth to skin for	...	20 minutes

Chronic Bronchitis

Jangli Pikvan (Ananttmul)		5 grs.
Liquorice root (Mulathi)		1 gr.
Ammonium Chloride	...	7 grs.
Kakad Singhi	...	5 "
Gum Babul	...	5 "
Common salt	...	2 grs.
Misce		

One powder to be taken twice a day.

Burns

Tilli Oil	...	1 ounces
Lime water	...	2 "

Apply locally

Cooling Lotion

Ammonia Chloride (Nawsagar)		2 drs.
Methylated Spirit	...	1 ounce
Water	...	10 ounces

Convulsions during labour

Borax (Sohaga)	...	10 grs.
Cinnamon (Dalchini)	...	10 "

Three times a day.

Cystitis

Isabgol seeds	...	2 drs.
Water	...	20 ounces

Boil for 10 minutes and strain, one ounce to be taken three times a day.

Delirium and Exhaustion

Musk (Kasturi)	...	1 gr.
Black pepper	...	1 "
Nutmeg (Jaiphal)	..	1 "
Mace (Jaipattri)	...	1 "
Long pepper (Pipul)	...	1 gr.

Make pill.

To be taken twice a day.

Carmanative Powder

Ginger (Sonth)	...	3 grs.
Black pepper (Kala Mirach)		3 "
Fennel fruit (Bari Sonf)		5 "
Black Salt (Kala Nimak)		10 grs.
Chebulic Myrobalans (Har)		10 "
Embelic Myrobalans (Awla)		10 "

One powder twice a day.

Chordi

Camphor	...	4 grains
Opium (Afim)	...	1/2 "

At bed time occasionally.

Chorea

Indian Spikenhead (Jatamansi)		2 drs.
Water	...	20 ounces

Macerate for 1/2 hour and strain, one ounce twice a day.

Conjunctivitis (Sore Eyes)

Alum (Phitkari)	...	5 grs.

Zinc Sulphate	2 "
Water	1 ounce

Two drops to be put twice a day.

Hepatitis

Ammonia Chloride (Nawsagar)	10 grs.
Potassium Nitrate (Shora)	10 "
Infusion Moringa (Shajna)	1 ounces

One ounce twice a day.

Hysteria

Aloes (Musabar)	5 Grs.
Asafoetida (Hing)	5 "
Camphor	2 "

One pill to be taken twice a day.

Laxative

Pulvis Senna leaves	5 grs.
Liquorice (Mulathi)	5 "
Sulphur (Gandhak)	3 "
Myrobalans (Har)	15"
Alu Bokara	10 "

Powder to be taken at bed time.

Pharyngitis

Bruised rind of Pomogranate	2 ounces
Cloves	1 dr.
Water	20 ounces

Boil for 20 minutes, and alum one drachm, as gargle.

Piles for external use only.

Opium (Afim)	30 grs.

Galls (Majuphal)	...	1 dr.
Simple Ointment	...	1 ounce

To be applied three times a day.

Laxative Powder for Piles

Kaladana	...	10 grs.
Sulphur	...	10 "

One powder every night.

For Prolapsed and Bleeding piles

Sulphate of Iron (Hera kas)		5 grs.
Common Salt	...	1 dr.
Water	...	2 ounces

As an enema twice a day.

Prickly Heat Powder

Camphor	...	2 grs.
Oxide of Zinc	...	1 dr.
Boracis	...	1 dr.
Starch	...	1 dr.
Vaseline	...	q. s.

To make an Ointment. To be applied twice a day.

Pruritus Vulvae

Borax (Sohaga)	...	4 dr.
Camphor water	...	8 ounces

For external application.

For Scabies

Sulphur (Gandhak)	...	1 dr.
Tilli Oil	...	1 ounces

For external use only, to be applied twice a day.

Ringworm

Boracis (Sohaga)	...	2 drs.
Vinegar (Sirka)	...	2 gus.
Sulphur	...	1 dr.

For external use only, to be applied twice a day.

Simple Ointment

Linseed Oil (Alsi oil)	...	4 ounces.
Suet (Charbi)	...	4 "
Wax	...	2 "

Basis for all Ointments.

Spermatorrhoea

Camphor (Kapur)	...	2 grs.
Extract Hyoscimus	...	1 gr.

One pill twice daily.

Synovitis (Painful Joints) for external use only

Aloes (Musabar)	...	4 drs.
Opium (Afim)	...	2 "
Rum	...	2 ounces

Warm down to a paste.

Tape-worm

Kamala	...	5 grs.
Powdered Butea Seeds (Palas bij)		5 "
Embolia Rebes (Babering)		5 "
Turpeth root (Pithora)		5 "
Honey	...	2 drs.

For one dose.

Tonic

Decoction of Sarsaparila root (Anantmul) ...	1 ounce.
Infusion Chiretta ...	1 "

To be taken twice a day.

Bitter Tonic

Infusion of Acorus root (Bach)	1 ounce
Infusion Chiretta ...	1 "

Tonic for Convalescence

Nim bark (Inner layer)...	2 ounce
Cloves ...	1 dr.
Water ...	30 ounce

Boil to ¼th and strain, one ounce twice a day.

Tonic Pill

Ferri Sulph (Rain) ...	2 grs.
Aloes (Musabar) ...	2 "
Cinnamon Powder (Dalchini)	4 "
Honey ...	q. s.

One pill to be taken twice a day.

Tympanitis

Asafoetida ...	20 ounces
Water ...	6 ounces

For an enema.

Ulcers

Turpentine Ointment

Oil of terpentine ...	1 ounce.
Sufed damar ...	1 dr.

Wax	...	4 drs.
Lard	...	4 drs.
Catechu (Katha)	...	1 ounce

Uterine Haemorrhage

Asoke bark	...	4 ounces
Water	...	20 "

Boil to ¼th and strain

One ounce twice a day.

Round-worm

Asafoetida (Hing)	...	3 grs.
Chiretta Powder	...	10 "

Powder to be taken at bed time.

For Cough Pneumonia

Juice of Tulsi leaves	...	2 drachms.
Juice of Mader leaves	...	10 drops.
Juice of garlic	...	40 "
Honey	...	4 drachms
Decoction of senna leaves..		20 drops
Aqua	...	1 oz.

For Diarrhoea with Blood

Bark of Apta tree	...	1 ounce
Bael fruit	...	1 "
Indra Java	...	20 grains
Juice of Tulsi leaves	...	3 drachms
Water	...	1 seer

Boil to 1/8th and strain.

One ounce to be taken twice a day.

Tulsi leaves	...	4 ounces
Water	...	20 "

Boil to 1/8th and strain.

Useful as diaphoretic.

Powdered dried Tulsi leaves		one ounce
Tannic Acid	...	one drachm
Boric Acid	...	two drachm
Bismath Carb	...	one ounce
Vekhand	...	one drachm

Useful in chronic ozena.

Powdered Tulsi leaves	...	one ounce
Ringni (Solanum Jacquinii)		two ounces
Vekhand	...	Four drachms
Water	...	Eight ounces
Tilli Oil	...	Fouri ounces

To be will pounded and evaporate the water and strain 3 or 4 drops to be put in the nose 3 or 4 times a day useful in dry chronic Ozoena.

Juice of Tulsi leaves	...	60 drops
Pudina Juice	...	15 drops
Black Pepper	...	30 grains
Myrrh	...	10 grains
Ginger Juice	...	60 drops
Lemon Juice	...	60 drops

To be taken twice a day.

Useful in Indigestion.

Powdered Bail fruit	...	grs. VI.

Pulvis Kino Co.	...	grs. I.
Sugar	...	II grs.
Misce		

To be taken twice a day. Useful in Diarrhoea among children.

Powdered Bail fruit	...	2 grs.
Bark of Bakul tree	...	1 "
Mayphal	...	2 "
Cloves	...	1 "
Sassafron Jaiphal	...	1 "
Kessar	...	½ "
Misce		

One powder to be taken twice a day.

Useful in chronic Diarrhoea of children between 5 and 10 years of age.

Vekhand	...	1 ounce
Kali myrrhe	...	1 dr.
Dhane	...	1 dr.
Aqua	...	20 ounces
Boil to	...	12 ounces

One tea spoonful in indigestion among children.

Vekhand Grains 20 as emetic acts as Ipecacuanha powder.

Garlic juice	...	4 drop
Hot water	...	1 ounce

In Whooping Cough among children 5 years of age twice a day.

Rheumatic liniment

Camphor	...	1 ounce

Oil of Turpentine ... 8 "

Soap water quantity sufficient.

For external use only.

Chronic Rheumatism

    Sulphur ... 2 ounces

    Nim Oil ... 20 "

Rub well into the joint. For external use only.

Purgative Powder

    Kaladana ... 10 grs.

    Rock Salt ... 10 "

    Rhubarb (Rewachini) ... 20 "

    Myrobalans (Har) ... 10 "

    Honey ... 1 dr.

    ft. Powder

to be taken at bed time.

For Piles with Constipation

    Chebulic Myrobalans Har   40 Grs

    Black Salt ... 20 "

    Beleric Myrobalans Beheda   30 "

    Embelic Myrobalans Awla   20 "

    Aniseed Sonf ... 20 "

    Ginger ... 10 "

    Senna leaves ... 10 "

60 grains of this to be taken in hot milk at bed time.

For Sore Nipples

For external use only.

    Borax (Sohaga) ... 60 grs.

| Simple Ointment | ... | 1 ounce |

For Chronic Malaria

Bonduck Seed Powder (Sagargota) 5 grs.
Gum ... q. s.
Make 12 pills of this
One pill twice a day

For Leucorrhoea. Astringent injection

Pomegranate fruit rind	...	3 ounces
Cloves	...	2 drachms
Water	...	2 pints

Boil for 15 minutes and add alum two drachms.
To be used twice a day as injection.

Laxative Powder

Rock Salt	...	5 grs.
Pulvis Senna leaves	...	10 grs.
Liquorice (Mulathi)	...	5 grs.
Sulphur (Gandhak)	...	5 grs.
Caraway (Jira)	...	5 grs.

Mix

One powder to be taken at bed time.

Shrir Sthan

From Susruta and Vagbhata.

Anatomy.

The following are the parts of the body skin:

कला Kala, धातु Dhatu, मल Mal, दोष Dosh, यकृत Yakrut (Liver), प्लिहा Spleen (Pleha), फुप्फुस Phuphus (Lungs), उराइक (Unduk), हृदय (Heart), आशय (Ashaya-stomach), आंतडी (Antadi-Intestines), स्रोतें (Sroten) openings.

कराडरा (big muscles), Kandara जालें (Jale), serous coverings, रज्जु (Rajju ligaments), शिवणी (Shewani sutures), हाडें (bones), सांधे (joints), स्नायु (snayu small muscles).

पेशी (Peshi), synovial membranes and covering मर्में (murme).

Vital spots, shira-blood vessels etc.

Skin.—Consists of seven layers.

According to Western science skin consists of cuticle which is non-vascular which is arranged in five layers. Another layer is of vascular connective tissue called corium or Cutis Vera. It is tough, flexible and elastic. Connective tissue consists of reticular and papillary layer.

Skin contains the peripheral endings of sensory nerves, blood vessels, sweat glands and lymphatics. Nails and hair are appendages of the skin.

कला (Kala): These are of seven kinds.

मांसधरा (Mansdhara): This is the whitish material seen on section of the muscle. In the muscles the blood vessels.

1. Lymphatics, muscle fibres and nerve intermingle.

2. रक्तधारा (Raktadhara): These are under the muscles and contain blood.

3. मेदोधरा (Medodhara): This is the fat of the body and the marrow of the bones.

4. श्लेमधरा (Shleshmdhara): This is the lubricating material found in the joints.

5. पुरीषधरा (Purishdhara): It is in the intestines. It separates the food juices from excreta.

6. मलधारा (Maldhara): It aids in the assimilation and absorption of food in the upper part of intestines.

7. शुक्रधरा (Shukradhara): This pervades the whole body आशय (Ashaya). वाताशय (Watashaya), nervous system पित्ताशय (Pitashay). The digestive system श्लेमाशय (shlemashay), lymphatic system, रक्ताशय (raktashay) circulatory system. Digestion in आमाशय (Amasaya), the digestion in the stomach पक्वाशय (Pakwashay), Intestinal tract. मुत्राशय (Mutrashay) bladder, and in the women there is uterus in addition.

Besides these the body contains यकृत (Yakrut), liver, प्लीहा (Pleha), spleen फुप्फुस (Fuffus) lungs. उराड़क (Unduk) Caecum, हृदय (Hridaya), heart, kidneys. मुत्रपिराड (Mutrapinds).

There are nine openings to the body. Two ears, two eyes, mouth, two nasal opening and urethral opening and in women there are two breasts in addition and vaginal opening.

Big muscles are 16 in number. In each leg they are (2) According to Western science they may be called gastroenemins and soleus. In each arm there are two, they are Biceps and Deltoid. In the neck there are four. According to Western science they are sterno-mustoid and Platysma on each side.

In the back they are four. Latassismus Dorsi and Trapezious on each side. All the muscles of the leg and hand are atached to the last portion of the bones at the nails.

Muscles of the back are attached to the bones lower down at the loins. Muscles that keep the neck erect are attached to the back part of the head. Muscles of the thigh are attached to the upper part of the hip bone and muscles of the arm are attached to the upper part of the bones of the shoulder. There are also nets of flesh, blood vessels, tendons and bones at the wrists and ankles.

There are also six intermingling of tissues made out of flesh, blood vessels, tendons and bones. They are at the elbows, knees, one in the neck and one in the generative organ. There are four big muscular tissues they are two external to the spine and two internal. They keep the muscles of the back in position.

शिवणी (Shivni) Sutures: They are seven, out of which five are in the head. According to Western science, they are the coronal suture, two squamosal sutures, one lambdoidal suture, one suture in the tongue and one in the generative organ between the corpus-spongiosum.

Joints are 14 in number. Two ankle joints, two knee joints, two hip joints, two at the wrist, two at the elbow, two at the shoulder, one at the back between the spine and sacrum and one between the head and spinal column. There are 300 bones in the body large and small.

According to Western science there are only 206. These are 3 bones on each finger and toes—so in both hands there are 30. There are ten bones on each feet, one bone at the ankle. In the leg there are two, in the thigh one and in the knee joint one, total 15 in each lower extremity.

In the loins there are five bones. In the chest on one side with cartilage there are 36.

According to Western science there are only 12 ribs. In the centre of the chest there are 8. There is only one in Western science and two collar bones. Ayurveda says that spinal column consists of 30 bones, while spinal column consists of 33 bones. In the neck there are 9 bones. While according to Western science there are seven bones. In the throat there are four bones, according to Western science there is one Hyoid bone. Nasal bones are considered to be three instead of two. All the bones of the head are taken to be one in Ayurveda while Western science divides. It consists of eight bones. Frontal, two temporal, one occipital, two parietal, one sphenoid and one ethamoid. All face bones are also considered to be one while there are several bones which go to make up the face such as superior-maxilla, nasal bones. Inferior maxilla on each side.

Western Anatomy says there are only 206 bones:

Axial skeleton

Vertebral column	26 bones	
Skull including face etc.	22	"
Hyoid bones	1	"
Ribs and sternum	25	"
Total	74	"
Upper extremities	64	
Lower extremities	62	
Total	126	
Auditory ossicles.	6	
Total	206	

Gray's Anatomy 1918 Edebon

Ayurveda divides the bones into five kinds. Flat such as teeth soft and flexible as found in children under one year. Curved as in ribs and hollow as found in thigh bones. Western science divides into long bones as seen in limbs, short as seen in hands, flat bones as seen in cranial bones and irregular bones as seen in spinal column. Bones support the white soft structure of the body. Joints, are divided into movable and immovable joints of hands and feet of the lower hip and shoulder and joint at the neck are movable. Ayurveda counts the number to be 210. Out of these, there are three joints in each of four toes and two in the last toe. Total 14. Besides there are three joints at the ankle knee and hip so also in the hands and one at wrist, elbow and shoulder, total 68. In the loins there are three, 24 in the spinal column, 24 in the chest and 8 in the middle. Eight in the neck, three in front of the throat etc., one in the nose, one in each eye, one in each cheek and ear, one at the lower lip one between the two eyebrows, five in the head etc. Western science divides also the joints into movable and immovable and slightly movable. Movable joints are divided into Hinge joint as joint between the fingers.

(b) Pivot joint.—As seen in Atlas joint.

(c) Condyloid.—Radio-carpal joint.

(d) Saddle joint.—Corpo-metacarpal joint of the thumb.

(e) Enar throsis.—Shoulder joint.

(f) Arthrodia.—Articular processes of vertibral.

Joints that are slightly movable. Tibio-fibular joint. Immovable articulation. Articulations of skull. Ayurveda divides the joints into eight kinds. कोर (Kor) such as phylangial joint, wrist, ankle, knee, elbow.

उडूखल (Udukhal) Hip, axilla, teeth etc. सामुदक (Samudag) Scapular joint and pelvic joint प्रत्तर (Paratar), vertibral joint तुन्नसेवनी (Tunna sevani) head bone joints.

वायसतुन्ड (Waysatunda) lower jaw joint. मंडल (Mandal) Orbital joint शखावर्त्त (Shankawart) Ear joint.

स्नायु (Snayu) muscles. They are 900 in number. Every toe has six muscles attached. In the feet there are 30. In the leg 30, knee 10, in the thingh 40, in the groin 10, total 150 in each lower extremity. In the hands fore-arm and arm there are the same number. In the abdomen and sides and chest 30. Head 34. They are 4 kinds. Long like tendon round flat and hollow.

According to Western science muscles are connected with the bones cartilages, ligaments and skin directly or indirectly. They are either long, broad or short and they considerably vary in the arrangement of their fibres. In some the fibres are parallel. These are quadrilateral muscles as in Thyro Hyodeus. In some they are slightly curved and they taper at the end. These are fusiform muscles. In some they arise from broad margin and convy to a tapering point as in temporal muscle. In some origin and insertion are not in the same plane as in Pectonus. In some the fibres are oblique and are attached to one side of the tendon as in Peroneus. These are unipernate and when they are attached to both sides of tendons they are called bipermate as in Rectus femoris.

In some the fibres are arranged in curved bundles as in Spincters.

Scalp	...	1
Eye-lids	...	3
Nose	...	5
Mouth	...	9
Mastication	...	4
	Total	22
	Superficial	3
Neck	Supra and Infra Thyroids	4
Upper	Anterior	4
extremity	Vertebrals	4
	Lateral vertebral	4
Trunk Deep		8

Sub-occipital	4
Thorax	8
Abdomen	6
Pelvis. Pelvis muscles posterior	4
Pelvic muscles	4
Perenium muscles	
Muscles of anal region	3
Uro-genital	5
Upper extremity, connecting the vertebral column.	5
Connecting thoracic wall	4
Shoulder muscles	6
Arm.	4
Fore-arm	5
Deep group	3
Back of fore-arm, superficial	7
Deep	5
Hand—Lateral volar	4
Medial	4
Intermediate	3
Lower extremity Muscles, of	
Illiac region	3
Muscles of thigh	7
Medial femoral muscles	5
Muscles of gluteal region	9

Post femoral muscles	3
Muscles of leg. Anterior crural Muscles.	4
	4
Deep group	4
Lateral crural group	2
Muscles of foot. Dorsal muscle	1
Planter. 1st layer	3
2nd layer	2
3rd layer	3
4th. " Dorsal	4
Plantar	3

So in each half of the body. There are 177 muscles or 354 on the whole body. To these add muscles of eye-balls and ear 14 in both eyes, 18 in both the ears extrinsic and intrinsic, total 386.

Peshi पेशी Fibrons Coverings—Ayurveda says these are 500 in number, covering the small muscular structures in each toe there are three. On the back of toes there are 10, in the feet 10, on the back of feet 10, near the ankle 10, leg 10, knee 5, thigh 20, groin 10, total 100. In each lower extremity so also in other leg and upper extremity.

Anus three, buttocks 5, bladder 2, stomach 5, umbilicus 1, upper part back 5, sides 6, chest 10, axilla and shoulder 7, heart and stomach 2, spleen, liver and caecum 6, neck 4, lower lip 8, throat 1, head 2, tongue 1, nose 2. In the females there are 20, around the breast, womb, and ovaries.

Murme मर्मे Vital spots they are 107, these are the spots where blood vessels, nerves, lymphatics and muscle fibres are close together.

1. Kshipra क्षिप्र: One inch between the toe and first meta-tarsal bone. It is half inch long. This is the place where extensor digitorus longus and flexor digitorum longus are attached to the toe.

2. तलहृदय (Tul-hridaya): In the middle of the Solar aspect of the foot. Here is planter arch and nerves close to each other.

3. कूर्च (Kurch): It is 2 inches above kshipra on the dorsum of the foot. Here are the tendons of extensor Hollusis Longus, Extensor Digitorum Longus and Tibialis Anticus are very close to each other.

4. कूर्चशीर (Kurchshir): This is about one inch long below the ankle on either side. Here also Tibialis Anticus and Extensor Longus Digitorum are in contact.

5. गुलफ (Gulph): It is below the ankle, 2 inches long on either side of the joint. Here on the inner side Post Tibial artery and vein, nerve, and tendons of the plantar muscles are in intimate contact and on the outside blood vessels and nerves and tendons of the extensor muscles of the foot.

6. इन्द्रबती (Indrabati): In the middle of the leg. This is the spot where there are Anti-Tibial and Post-Tibial arteries, nerves and veins close to each other. Injury to this brings on death by haemorrhage.

Janu जानु: It is situated in the knee joint. Injury to this causes lameness.

Ani आनि: It is situated three inches above the knee. It is the place of quadriceps extensor muscle.

Urvi ऊर्वी: This is the place in the middle of the thigh on its inner side. It is the site of the femoral artery, the spot where it passes through Adductor magnus to become popliteal artery. Injury to this causes death through haemorrhage.

Lohitaksh लोहिताक्षः This is the middle of popar's ligament, a spot mid-way in the groin. This is the place where Illiac artery comes into the thigh and becomes femoral. Injury to this causes death through haemorrhage.

Witap विटपः This is between the inner side of the groin and testis about an inch long. Injury to this causes atrophy of testis. This is the place were the spermatic cord containing Vas deferans and other structures traverse the Inguinal canal to the abdominal ring.

In the hand, there is (Kshipra) क्षिप्र a vital spot between the thumb and Index finger, a place where the opponens Polisis. Abductor Polisis and Flexor Brevis Polisis and Flexor Sublimis Polisis and Flexor. Longus Digitorum meet.

Tul-Rhidrya तलहृदयः This represents the middle of the palm. Here is the palmer arch, nerves and muscles close together.

Kurch कुर्चः It is 2 inches above Kshipra. Here are the tendons of Flexor-Digitorum-Sublimis, Digital arteries and nerves.

कूर्चशीर (Kurchshir): This is 1" below the wrist. It is the place where there are Flexor and Extensor tendons of the muscles, pronators, Radial and Ulnar nerves, arteries and veins.

इन्द्रवती (Indrabati): It is in the middle of the forearm.

This is the place where there are Radial arteries, veins and nerves and layer of superficial muscles of the forearm.

मनिबन्ध (Manibandh): It is two inches below the elbow. There are radial and ulnar arteries.

कूर्पुर (Kurpur): This is elbow joint the place where the brachial artery divides into ulnar and radial and median nerve.

ऊर्वी (Urwi): This is in the middle of the arm on its inner side. The place where median nerve lies in front of brachial artery.

लोहिताक्ष (Lohitaksh.): A place near the lower border of axilla below the border of Pectoralis major, a place where axillary artery becomes brachial. Injury to it causes death by haemorrhage.

कक्षधर (Kashdhar): It is the place where subclavian artery emerges and becomes the axillary artery. A place in the lower third of axilla about its upper third.

Rectum. गुद (Gud): Injury to this is attended with serious consequences and so also the bladder बस्तिमर्म (Bastimurma).

Umbilicus नाभी (Nabhi) is another vital spot.

Rhidaya हृदय (heart) is in the chest. There are two vital spots about one inch below the nipples. This is the place of Aortic arch and Pulmonary arteries on the right and one inch above the nipple is another vital spot on each side, because below it are important blood vessels opening into the heart. These are स्थनरोहित (Sthanrohit).

अपलाप (Aplap): This spot is above the middle third of collar bone. There is the subclavian artery on each side.

अपस्तंथ (Apasthamb): The spot is close to the root of the neck. These are the right and left common carotid arteries.

Back

कटिक तरूण (Katiq tarum): The spot is on either side of the end of the vertibral column. This is the place where important nerves come out.

कुकुंदर (Kukundar): This spot is to the outer side of the fist. There are the sacro-Illiac joint on each side.

नितम्ब (Nitamb): This is the part where sacral plexus is situated. This is just below the lumber region.

पार्श्वसन्धी (Parashwa sandhi.): The spot is over the kidney region on each side.

बृहती (Bruhati): The spot is in the line of the nipple to the vertebral column. On the right side is the liver and on the left is the heart.

अंसफलक (Aunsphalak): Spot is the upper part of the back in the line with the shoulder joint. There is the Brachial plexus.

अस (As): This is the spot between the top of the shoulder and neck and back of the shoulder blade. Injury to this causes impairment of shoulder. There are Deltoid Trapezeous and other shoulder muscles.

Vital spots in the neck and above

घमनी (Dhamani): These are two spots on each side of Trachia in the neck. There are the superior and inferior laryngeal nerves branches of vagus on each side. They cause loss of voice, loss of taste etc.

मातृका (Matruka): There are four blood vessels on each side of the neck. These are carotid arteries and vein.

कृकाटिका (Krukatica): This is the joint between the head and neck, that is between Atlas fist, cervical vertibra and base of the bone.

विधुर (Vidhur): A spot behind the ear on each side. Injury causes deafness. These are the mastoid processes of temporal bone.

फणा (Fana): Spot inside the nose. Injury to this causes abolition of smell. These are the olfactory nerves.

अंपाग (Apang.) The spot near the outer side of the eye on each side. Injury to this causes defective vision and loss of sight.

Here are the branches of Opthalmic, first division of fifth nerve and muscular branches of temporal nerve of seventh or facial nerve.

आवर्त (Awart.): The spot is above the eye-brow on the inner side of each side. Injury to this causes some defect in the eyes because there are Supra-Trochlear and Infra-Trochlear branches of Frontal nerves, a branch of Opthalmic nerve.

शंख (Shankh): The spot is the articulation of Temporal bone to the frontal bone. A blow or injury on it causes instantaneous death.

उत्क्षेप (Utkshep): The spot is the top of the head. This is vertex of the skull. Injury to this causes fainting.

स्थपनी (Sthapani): Is the spot between the two eye brows. Front of the brain is closer to the skull in this part. Injury to this causes unconsciousness.

सामन्त (Samanth): These are the five articulations in the skull.

शृंगाटक (Shrungatak): These spots are four and are close to arterial circle of Willis.

This is situated in the subarachnoid space at the base of the brain and encloses the optic chiasma and structures in the inter peduncular fossa. In front the two anterior cerebral arteries each of which is joined to the internal carotid artery of the same side by the posterior communicating artery. Injury, to this region is always fatal.

Adhipati अधिपति: The spot is the middle of the cortex of the brain indicated in the skull slightly to the outer side of the top of the head on each side. Injury to this causes instantaneously death.

Shira शिरा Blood vessels and nerves in the body.

They are divided into four kinds (Watwah) वातावह that is nerves. They are yellowish brown, (Pittwaha) पित्तवाह are blue i.e. veins and (Kuffwah) कफ़वाह are white and tough that is they are lymphatics and (Rakat-wah) रक्तवाह are red. They carry blood i.e. arteries. In each lower and upper extremity there are 100 of these kinds.

Arteries

Sole of the feet. Lateral plantar artery.

Ankle–Anterior Posterior Tibial Leg–Anterior Tibial, Posterior Tibial and Peroneal.

Knee Joint–Popletcal.

Thigh–Femoral and Profunda.

These are principal arteries according to Western science principal superficial veins in the lower extremity.

1. Dorsal digital and metatarsal veins.
2. Dorsal venous arch.
3. Planter cutaneous venous arch.
4. Plantar cutaneous venous network.
5. Great saphenous vein.
6. Small saphenous vein.

Deep Veins

1. Deep plantar cutaneous and metatarsal veins.
2. Deep plantar venous arch.
3. Posterior tibial veins.

4. Anterior tibial veins.
5. Popletial vein.
6. Femoral vein.

Lymphatics

1. Superficial lymphatic vessels medial. They accompany the great and small saphenous vein. 2. Anterior tibial. 3. Posterior tibial 4. Peroneal.

Nerves–Medial plantar and lateral and lateral plantar the branches of internal popliteal nerve.

Tibial.
2. Internal Popliteal nerve.
3. Common peroneal nerve.
4. Sciatic nerve in the thigh.
5. Femoral nerve.
6. Saphenous nerve.

Upper extremity

Principal arteries.—1. Axillary artery. 2. Brachial in the arm. 3. Radial and ulnar in the forearm. 4 Inter osseons. 5. Superficial and deep palmar arteries in the hand. 6. Deep volar arch in the back of the hand.

Principal veins

1. Dorsal digital and metacarpal veins.
2. Posterior volar digital veins.
3. Cephalic vein.
4. Basilic vein.
5. Median cephalic and median basilic veins.
6. Deep volar metacarpal veins
7. Venacometes of radial and ulnar arteries.

8. Brachial veins on either side of the artery.
9. Axillary vein.

Lymphatics

Superficial lymphatic vessels follow the course of cephalic, median ,brachial and basilic veins. Deep lymphatic vessels accompany the course of radial ulnar, volar, inter osseons arteries.

Nerves

Axillary nerve, musculo-cutansous, musculo-spiral, median, ulnar and radial and posterior, interosseons and palmer and dorsal branches of radial and ulnar nerves.

Abdomen

Principal arteries, 1. Abdominal Aorta, 2. Right and left common Illiacs, 3. Caeliac, 4. Superior and inferior messenteric, 5. Renal, 6. Testicular in the male and ovarian in the female, 7. Inferior phrenic, 8. Lumbar, 9. Middle sacral.

Veins

1. Inferior venacava, 2. Lumbar veins, 3. Testicular in the males and ovarian in females, 4. Renal, 5. Inferior phrenic, 6. Hepatic veins, 7. Portal vein formed of spleenic, superior Messenteric, coronary, gastric, csytic, and Parumbelical.

Nerves: Sacral and lumbar plexuses, lumbar plexus gives rise to Illio-Inguinal, Illio-Hypogastric, genito femoral, femoral obturator and lumbo-sacral nerves.

Sacral plexus gives rise to superior gluteal. Inferior gluteal sciatic, Pudendal and Ano-coccegeal.

Chest: Principal arteries are: 1. Aortic arch, 2. Innominate artery, 3. Left common carotid, 4. Right and left subclavian, 5. Right and left pulmonary arteries, 6. Internal mammary arteries.

Veins: 1. Right and left pulmonary veins 2. superior venacava 3. Inferior vena cava, 4. Right Innominate vein, 5. Left common carotid vein, 6. Right and left pulmonary veins.

Lymphatic vessels: Thoracic duct and its tributaries, Posterior Intercostal vessels of seven intercostal spaces, and lymphatic vessels from the upper five intercostal spaces, 2. Lymphatic vessels of the heart, 3. Lymphatic vessels of the lungs and pleura, 4. Lymphatic vessels of Thymus and aesophagus, 5. Lymphatic vessels of the diaphragm and intercostal arteries, 6. Lymphatic vessels of the breasts and other superficial lymphatic vessels.

Neck Principal arteries, 1. Right and left common carotids, 2. Right and left subclavian, 3. External and Internal carotids on each side, 4. Superior Thyroid, 5. Lingnal, 6. External maxillary, 7. Occipital, 8. Posterior Auricular, 9. Temporal and Internal maxillary.

Veins: 1. External jugular, 2. Anterior and Internal and Posterior jugular, 3. Vertebral, 4. Lingual, 5. Thyroid, 6. Vertebral, 7. Right and left Internal jugular vein.

Lymphatics: 1. Superficial lymphatic vessels of the neck, 2. Lymphatic vessels from the Larynx and thyroid gland.

Nerves: 1. Hypoglossal, 2. Lingual, 3. Vagus, 4. Glassopharingeal, 5. Phrenic, 6. Accessary, 7. Cervical branches of cervical plexus.

Head and face: Principal arteries.

1. Facial, 2. Lingual, 3. Temporal, 4. Post auricutar on either side, 5. Opthalmic and in the head vertebral and temporal.

Veins: 1. Lingual, 2. Facial, 3. Temporal, 4. Posterior auricular, 5. Vertebral.

Lymphatics: 1. Lymphatic vessels of the scalp, 2. Lymphatic vessels of the ear and nose and mouth, 3. Lymphatic vessels of tonsils and tongue.

Nerves: Lingual, glossopharyngeal, facial nerves, opthalmic division of fifth nerve.

Brain: Principal arteries.

1. Anterior cerebral, 2. Middle cerebral, 3. Posterior communicating. 4. Anterior choroidal, 5. Basilar and Internal carotid.

Veins: 1. External cerebral veins, 2. Basal veins, 3. Cerebellar veins, 4. Five venons sinuses of duramater, 5. Two cavernous sinus, 6. Two intra cavernous, 7. Two superior petrosal and two inferior, 8. Basilar plexus, 9. middle Meningeal vein.

Lymphatics: 1. Superficial lymphatics of the scalp.

2. Lymphatic vessel from ears and face and mouth.

3. Lymphatic vessels from tonsils and nose.

4. Lymphatic vessels from tongue.

Nerves: 1. Olfactory, 2. Optic, 3. Oculomotor, 4. Trochlear, 5. Trigeminal, 6. Abducent, 7. Facial, 8. Auditory, 9. Glosopharyngeal, 10. Vagus, 11. Accessory, 12. Hypoglossal.

According to Ayruveda, out of these four those that carry (Vat) वात are yellowish brown in colour and they are probably nerves. There are 25 nerves in each lower and upper extremity, in abdomen 34, loins 8, back 6, stomach 6, sides on each side 2, chest 10, and in the neck 14, ears two, in each 9, in the tongue, nose 6, eyes four, in each. Total 175. The same number is of arteries, veins and lymphatics. The principal nerves in the body are 10 arteries, 10 veins, and lymphatics 10 and others are the branches of these.

Veins:

Lymphatics: 1. Superficial lymphatic vessels that follow the course of superficial blood vessels and the deep vessels. 2. Lymphatic vessels of the stomach and Intestines, 3. Lymphatic vessels of liver, Pancreas, kidney, bladder, 4. Lymphatic vessels of reproductive organs, 5. Origin of Thoracic duct.

Foetal Life In Ayurveda

Soul influenced by actions of past life gets united in the common cell formed by the union of male and female cells at the time of conception, as fire is produced by friction.

बीजात्मकैर्महा भूतैः सूक्ष्मैः सत्वानु गैश्चसः ।
मातुश्च आहार रसजैः क्रमात्कुक्षौ विवर्धते । ।
वाग्भट शरीर स्थान अध्याय १ श्लोक ४

Elements that exist in semen of men and ovum of women and elements that come along with soul and elements that are produced from the diet and blood of the mother nourish and develop the foetus.

Soul is invisible while combining with the cell formed after fertilization which consists in the union of sperm cell with the mature ovum just as ray of sun light from condensed glass remains invisible while passing to a dried cow dung cake.

कारणानु विधायित्वात् कार्यीणां तत्स्वभावता ।
नाना योन्या कृतीः सत्वोधत्ते ऊतो द्रुत लोहवत् । ।
वाग्भट अध्याय १ श्लोक ४

Result of action being dependent on cause, there is similarity between cause and effect just as liquid iron formed after heating assumes different forms when put in different moulds in the same way souls also assumes different froms.

If the elements existing in the sperm cell are in excess to the elements in the female cell at the time of conception it gives rise to male, if female elements predominate then a female child and when they are of equal proportion then a neuter. If the elements of sperm or ovum cells are divided by वायु (Vayu) by nervous elements of husband and wife at the time of conception then it gives rise to more than one foetus according as the elements of male or female predominate and when the nerve element वात (Vat) is in disordered condition, then it gives rise to monsters.

Females have menstrual flow every month and lasts for 3 days. Best age of conception is that of 20 years of the male and 16 years of female.

Semen which is disordered by वात (Vat) पित्त (Pitt) or कफ (Kuff) or by other diseases does not possess the property of conception. Semen which is white, thick, sticky and excessive is fit for conception, signs of womanhood. The girls gets shy breasts become bigger and menstrual flow occurs every month and lasts for 3 or 4 days. In menstrual period woman should remain on light diet and sleep on hard bed and take aperient food.

Signs of conception, complete satisfaction, slight heaviness in the womb, palpitation with fainting, thirst and coldness of the skin united cell becomes visible in 7 days in the womb.

If the woman desires a male child she should take good nourishing food and tonics.

Pregnant woman should give up hard exercise. Untimely going to bed sitting on hard ground, emotional feelings such as fright, anger, fasting, unsuitable food, alcohol and meat eating.

In the second month the feetus becomes solid and round or semi-circular. When the feetus becomes visible the womb, is enlarged and feels heavy. Mother gets vomiting, tastelessness, salivation, attacks of fainting, or giddiness, desire to eat acid things, enlargement of breast and pigmentation around the nipples, swelling of the feet, headache and burning of the hands and feet.

In the third month of pregnancy, two hands two feet and head become distinguishable, and feetus is connected by one hollow tube which carries the blood.

Fourth month, All parts become visible and in the fifth heart begins to beat.

Sixth month, muscles, arteries, hair, colour, nails and skin become visible.

Seventh month, all the limbs of the feetus get developed. Eight month, these parts get fatty and develop nails and hair get longer.

In the ninth feetus becomes fully developed and the woman becomes fit for delivery.

Approaching signs of delivery:

Thinness, feeling of exhaustion, heaviness in the loins, tastelessness in the mouth, salivation. Frequency of micturition. Pains in the joints, abdomen and back. Pains in the womb and discharge. After this, there is discharge of watery fluid from the womb. At the time of delivery the woman should be on her back and her womb should be massaged .... This .. promotes foetus to come down.

Labour: In the beginning she should be given light food and she should be made to walk about when the womb pains become severe she should be put on bed and she should hold her breath and lean down and after the child is born expression of placenta वार (War) is carried out by kneading the uterus.

It the foetus gets obstructed the root of सोना चाफ (Sonachampa) tree of yellow flower should be given in her hand and feet to hold. Her body should be shaken with both hands or pressed at the buttocks. Her womb should be fomented with bitter लौकी ((Lowki) leaves of शिरस (shiras) or decoction of तुलसी पत्र and Tulsee leaves one ounce each in 8 ounces of water boiled to 1/8th, one ounce may be given every fourth hour to promote uterine pains or douche of Badishope, asafoetida and rock salt one teaspoon full each in 32 ounces of hot water is also useful, or an intelligent nurse should remove her nails and remove placenta.

After the placenta, child should be cleaned thoroughly and mother given light food.

Obstructed Labour

मूढ गर्भ (Mudh garbh) when the hand, feet or head remains in the transverse position at the os or both the hands and feet it is called विष्कंभ मूढगर्भ (Vighkamph mudhgarbh.) All these are required to be removed by instruments when any limb of the faetus is not in the direct line for exit. It should be brought in that line earlier by turning or by pressure over the womb and then pulled out. In certain cases when the foetus is unable to come out, head bones are rquired to be broken and then foetus removed by pulling axilla or lip. In shoulder presentation the faetus is removed by instrument called गर्भशंकु (garbh shanku) either by cutting the arm and then pulling or evisceration. It is required to be divided. After the foetus is removed the mother should be given hot bath and cotton emersed in oil should be put at the mouth of the womb. If the woman is dead during labour then foetus should be removed by incision in the abdomen and through the womb.

According to Western science, fertilization consists in the union of the Spermatozoan with the mature ovum.

Fertilization of the human ovum takes place in the lateral or ampullary part of the uterine tube. It is then conveyed along the tube to the cavity of uterus in 7 or 8 days when it undergoes segmentation. If it is arrested in the tube tubal pregnancy occurs or if it falls in the abdominal cavity then abdominal pregnancy. Under normal condition only one spermatozoa enters the yolk and occasionally two which give rise to monstrosity.

Growth of the Ovum.

1st month — Length 1/12th inch, embryo is nourished by osmosis. At the end of fourth week the ovum is about the size of pigeon's egg and length 1/3 inch.

2nd month — The ovum is about the size of hen's egg, and embryo 1¼th inch long and 240 grams in weight.

3rd month — Ovum is about the size of orange, weighs 85 grams. Placenta formed. Points of ossification in bones.

4th month — Foetus is about 5 inches and 7½ ounces in weight. Sexual organs distinct.

5th month — Foetus 10 inches and weight 454 grams. Hair appearing, Vernix caseosa present.

6th month — Foetus 12 inches long, weight 2½ pounds. Eyebrows and lashes appearing.

7th month — Foetus is 14 inches long and weighs 3 pounds. Pupillary membrane present, and in the male foetus the testes have reached the Inguinal-canal.

8th month — Foetus is 16 inches long and weighs 4½ pounds, fat present, pupillary membrane slightly present, and it is disappearing.

9th month — Foetus is 18 inches long, weighs 5 pounds, the nails have not quite reached the ends of the fingers.

The full terms ovum-consists of Chorian, Amnion, Placenta, Umbilical cord, Liqr-Amnii; and foetus.

Phenomenon of Pregnancy

    1. Changes in the uterus, vagina, fallopian tubes, and ovaries.

    2. Changes in the pelvic joints.

    3. Changes in the breasts.

    4. Pigmentation.

    5. Effects in urinary and digestive systems.

Diagnosis of Pregnancy

    1. Cessation of menses. 2. Morning sickness. 3. Quickening. 4. Salivation. 5. Enlargement of Breasts 6. Uterine soufle. 7. Quickening and foetal heart sounds.

Mechanism of Labour

    1. Descent, 2. Flexion (vertex) or extension face. No corresponding movement in pelvic presentation, 3. Internal Rotation, 4. Extension (vertex), Flexion (face), Spinal latero-flexion (pelvic), 5. External Rotation.

Management of Labour

    Preparation for labour—Room should be clean and well lighted. Enema at the beginning of labour, and draw off urine.

    At the beginning when the contractions are few, she should have some occupation and let the patient walk about and do not interfere. Second stage begins with the dilatation of os and ends with the birth of the child. Put the patient in such a position as she can best lean-down, and as soon as head appears in the vulva, the indication is to obtain slow delivery of the head and to ensure that the smallest possible diameter distends the pereneutium. After the child is born the patient is turned on her back and hand is placed on the womb. As soon as the cord has ceased pulsating it is tied and the child separated. Empty the bladder and wait. Keep the hand in the womb till the placenta comes out and then sterilized dressings are applied to the vulva and ergot one drachm given.

Chapter XII

Diet in Ayurveda From सुश्रुत Sushruta

शालिवर्ग—Shaliwarg.

Rice grains are easy to boil and tend to increase slightly Pitt & Kuff (पित्त और कफ़).

Red rice is slightly diuretic, and easily digestible.

देवभात (Dewbhat), वरया (Warya), राळे (Rale), increase पित्त (Pitt) and diminish कफ़ (Kuff).

मुग (Mug), वाटाणे Peas, मसुर (Masur) gram हरभरे और मटर Mutar.

They increase वात (Vat), and diminish पित्त और कफ़ (Pitt and Kuff). Out of these मुग (Mug) is easily digestible.

उडद (Urad) is heavy and increases urine and milk and कफ Kuff.

चवली (Chawli) Kulith, diminish वात (Vat) and कफ Kuff.

तील (Til): They are tonic but increase कफ़ Kuff.

Black variety is the best.

जवस (Linseed): It is demulcent, allays thirst and aperient.

गहु (Wheat): It is a strengthening food.

मोहरी (Mustard): It is stimulant and diminishes कफ़. Kuff and वात (Vat).

मांसवर्ग meat of various kind.

Meat of black buck and deer: It is tonic and strengthening food.

कोंबडी Foul or chickem: Is light to digest and useful in consumption.

मोर Peacock: It is a very light food to digest and strengthening food and good for brain.

कबुतर Pigeon: It is a very light food to digest and useful in bowel complaints and in typhoid fevers.

बकरा Mutton: It is strengthening to the muscles but little heavy to digest.

गाय Cow: It is slightly heavier than mutton to digest and also a strengthening food. Soup is usually given in Typhoid cases.

डुकर Pig: It is tonic and promotes perspiration.

कासव Tortoise meat is heavy to digest but it is very strengthening.

मासा Fish: They are divided into salt water and fresh water fish. They are light to digest and are brain tonic and more strengthening.

Sea fishes are more strengthening.

All dry decomposed, or poisoned or cut with poisoned or rusty knife, meat of old, lean or very young animals living on bad food is not fit to eat.

Meat of females in animals, meat of young ones in birds are more suitable for digestion. Most of mid part of all animals is heavy to digest, among males the front portion and among females the back portion meat of those birds that live on fruits is easily digestible. Meat of those birds who eat fish increase Pitt पित्त and those that live on grain is good to digest and diminish वात Vat. Meat of the part near the liver is more nourishing and easily digestible.

डालींब Pomegranate, आंवला Awala, बोर Ber, कवठ Kawath, Mahalung mangoe, महालुंग Karwand, करवंद, (चारोळी the seed of Achar). (नारींग oranges, lemons), कोकम Kokum Lotus seeds, Tamarind फणस jack fruit. They are acid heavy to digest and increase कफ Kuff.

डालिंब Pomegranate allays पित्त Pitt and appetiser, Awla आंवला allays Pitt and Kuff and is Stomachic. Ber बोर are slightly aperient. कवठ (Kethu) stomachic and allays thirst.

महालुंग Mahalung: Appetiser and is good in dyspepsia,

आंबा Mango, slightly aperient and strengthening food.

करवंद Karwand: Allays thirst, stimulates saliva and increases appetite.

चारोळी Achar seed: Strengthening food.

अननस Ananas, stomachic and diminishes Vat वात.

कोकम Kokumb: Appetiser and stomachic.

चिंच Tamarind: Aperient and allays thirst.

नारंगी Orange: Stimulant to the heart, appetiser, slightly aperient and stomachic.

Lemon: Allays thirst, stomach ache, vomiting and stomachic it diminishes (Pitt) पित्त.

Phanas फनस: It is strengthening and aperient. Heavy to digest.

Jambul जांबुळ: Astringent and diminishes the (Vat) वात and (Kuff) कफ.

Khirani खिरणी: They are heavy to digest.

Bakul वकुल: Astringent. They strengthen the teeth.

Fige अंजीर. Aperient and tonic..

Kamalkand कमलकंद. Tonic and strengthening food and stimulant to the heart.

Bel Phal बेलफल. Aperient, demulcent and strengthening and appetiser.

Tondale तोंडलें: Increases milk.

Palm fruit ताडगोळा: Diuretic, heavy to digest and tonic.

Plantain केळी: Heavy to digest but strengthening food.

Cocoanut नारयळ. Aperient and strengthening food.

Grapes द्राक्षें: Aperient and allays thirst given in consumption.

Khajur खजुर: Stimulant to the heart strengthening food.

Almonds अक्रोड (Akrod), (Pista) पिस्ता: They are all heavy to digest but improve the blood.

Rai Awala राय आंवला: Stomachic, stimulant to the heart and increases the flow of saliva.

Bhonkar भोंकर: It is demulcent.

Biba बिबा: The fruit of marking nut is astringent and strengthening food.

Karanj करंज, (Palas) पलास and (Kadu Nimb) कडूनिंब fruits: They are against worms.

Wawding वावडींग: It expells the worms and tonic.

Hirda हिरडा: Appetiser and aperient.

Behada बेहडा: Appetiser, aperient and expels worms.

Supari सुपारी. Promotes salivation.

Camphor कापुर. Allays thirst and stomachic.

Vegetables

Koholla Pumpkin कोहला: It diminishes Pitt and tonic.

Kalingad कलिंगड: It increases (Kuff) कफ and (Vat) वात. Heavy to digest and promotes diarrhoea.

Cucumbar काकडी: Heavy to digest promotes diarrhoea.

Green Pipeli पिंपळी, and (Mire) मिरे are stomachic and diminish (Pitt) पित्त.

Punarnawa पुनर्नवा: It diminishes (Kuff) कफ and (Vat) वात often used in dropsy and inflammations.

Raddish मुल: It is stomachic and stimulant to the heart.

Garlic लसुण: It is stomachic and stimulant and aids in digestion used in consumption.

Onion कांदा: Heavy to digest. It increases Pitt (पित्त). Vegetable of (Rajgira) राजगिरा, (Tandurja) तांदुरजा, (Methi) मेथी and चाकवात Chakwat. Are diuretic and increase to some extent (Vat) वात and (Pitt) पित्त.

Padwal पडवळ, Brinjals वांगी (Karle) कालें, दोडके Dodke: They are stimulant to the heart and digestive.

Ambad choka आंवड चुका: Astringent used in diarrhoea.

Nadishak नाडीशाक अंलु: Alu astringent and appetiser, useful in diarrhoea.

Ghol घोळ: It is aperient and stomachic.

Leaves of gram and peas: Aperient.

Betal leaves पान: Stimulant and appetiser.

पुष्प वर्ग Flowers

Flowers of जाई (Jai) and जुई (Jui): They diminish (Pitt) पित्त by their smell. Not to be eaten.

Bakul बकुल and गुलाब (Rose) are stimulant to the heart. Champa चंपा: It diminishes Kuff.

Mushrooms: They are diuretic and so also young bamboo leaves. They increase (Vat) वात.

कंद वर्ग Root Vegetables

Bhui Kohla ground pumpkin. भुय कोहला

Shingade शिंगाडे, (Ratali) रताळी they are sweet, easy to digest and increase milk and tonic and strengthening food.

कृतान्नवर्ग (Krutan warg) *Cooked food.*

Ripe mangoes are laxative and tonic. Ripe bale fruit. astringent. Useful in diarrhoea and dysentery.

Jack fruit: Seed is excellent food.

Tamarin water: Aperient and allays thirst. Plantains very nutritions but difficult to digest.

Cocoanut: Nutritious. Is useful in the diet of diabetes Wall nut Nutritious food.

Western science on diet lays great stress on milk and its preparations. It is valuable in acute febrile conditions and in irritable stomach, given with soda water or peptonized in vomiting. It is combined with lime water in catarrh and ulceration of small Intestines. It is forbidden in obesity, gout, gravel, diabetes. It is the best diet in Acute nephrbites, arterio-selerosis and high arterial pressure. It is sterilized by being subjected to a temperature of steam for 30 minutes to 60.

Whey contains 25 p.c. of nitrogenous matter all the sugar and salts of milk. It is one of the substitutes for human milk given to artificially fed infants. $3\frac{1}{2}$ ounce sherry to one pint of milk is white wine whey. Butter milk contains proteins, sugar and salts of milk and 1/3rd of original fat, useful in Intestinal toxaemia.

Cream: Is given when fats are contraindicated.

Eggs: Given in protracted fevers, albumen water is given in persistent vomiting.

Meat: It is easily digested in stomach and small intestines, tinned meat, raw or slightly cooked is given in diabetes. It is forbidden in chronic intestitial nephritis, high blood pressure, gout, arterial sclerosis, but a liberal protein diet reduces oedema in parenchymatous nephritis. Thymus and Pancreas, brains, liver etc. Are easily digested and given in feeble stomachs. They are forbidden in chronic interstitial nephritis and high blood pressure.

Chicken: Diet is given to convalescent patients as they contain more protein and less fat.

Fish: Is less nitrogenous. Boiled fish is the most easily digested.

Beef: Mutton or chicken contain 12 p.c. solids with gelatin and stimulant salts. They are unsuitable in diarrhoea unless this is traced to infected milk.

Meat juice: Is valuable to exhaustion in intolerant stomach.

Bread: Starches such as rice, Arrowroot, sago, Tapioka, corn flour and potatoes. These are cabro-hydrates. They are the principal elements of semi-solid diet in returning appetite and digestion from acute fevers. Peptonized bread, gruel, pancreatized food, malt extract, baked flour and sugar are useful in structural affections of stomach and intestines. Pastry is unsuitable in gastric catarrh with dilatation and fermentation and cardiac and respiratory diseases. Boiled rice eaten with chicken or fish is useful in some intestinal diseases.

Brown or white meal breads and oatmeal stimulate peristalsis in chronic constipation. Carbohydrates are forbidden in obesity and diabetes. They are useful in chronic interstitial nephritis.

Fats and oils: Butter, cream, yolk of egg, codliver oil etc. They are nutritious and are useful in all wasting diseases such as Tuberculosis, Osteo-arthritis, Neurestenia, Renal disease. They are forbidden in obesity.

Green or other vegetables: They have a mild aperient action in constipation and they aggravate diarrhoea. They also cause flatulent, indigestion in the stomach and bowels. They are good substitutes for potatoes in diabetes and obesity gout, and Bright's disease. Rhubarb and Tomatoes are unsuitable in oxaluria.

Fruit: It is best eaten in the morning useful in febrile states and to supplement the diet in chronic nephritis, grapes cause flatulence.

Figs and prunes are useful in constipation.

Orange and lemon are antiscorbutic.

Food is given perrectum: As nutrient enemata and nutrient suppositories. It consists of milk alone or milk and egg. Enemata of milk, gruel, eggs or preparations of meat are given pancreatized.

In every case rectum is washed out with warm water atleast once daily.

Nutrient suppositories 30 to 60 grams of peptonized milk. These are employed in structural disease's or excessive irritability of stomach with vomiting and in aesophaegeal obstruction.

Shingadas शिंगाडे are astringent.

Suran सुरण: Heavy for digestion. Astringent.

Ransuran, रानसुरन increases Pitt (पित्त).

Lotus kand. कुमुद (Kumud) allays palpitation of the heart.

लवण वर्ग Salts

Rock salt, सैन्धव (Sandhaw), sea salt बिडलोण (Beedlone), पादेलोण (Padelone), रोमक (Romak), सांभरकीठ (Sambharmit) salt from the lake—they are aperient and diuretic.

Rock salt: It is digestive and stimulant. Sea salt in large doses is emetic and allays colic. Beedlone is stomachic and stimulant. Padelone, is stimulant, stomachic and useful in stomach colic. Romak is diuretic and aperient.

Jawakhar जवाखार (Sajjikhar सज्जीखार) are stimulant and promote the flow of saliva and aid digestion. (Takan khar) टाकणखार is astringent and used against inflammation.

Metals

Gold, its preparations are considered to be tonic and destroy poison. Silver and its preparations are astringent tonic and reduce (Vat) वात and (Pitt) पित्त. Copper is astringent and germicide, iron and its preparations are tonic and improve the quality of blood and astringent. Zinc and lead are astringent. Pearls and its preparations are also tonic and astringent. Among all the grains साठेतांदुल (Sathetandul) rice सातु (Satu), गहु (Gahu) wheat, लालतांदुल (Laltandul) Red rice, मुग (Mung), तुवर (Tuar) मसुर Masur are the best. Meats of pigeons, buck, peacock and tortoise, chicken tender mutton are the best.

Pomegranate, awala, grapes, dates, khirani, mahlung, orange, lemon, mango are the best.

Among vegetables चाकवत (chakwat, radish methi, math alu, are good. Cow's milk is the best and also her ghee for medical purposes. Rock salt Pipeli and ginger are good digestive. Among sweets honey is the best and also cane sugar. Old rice is very light for digestion.

Honey

New honey is strengthening and aperient year old reduces the fat and astringent. It should not be eaten with hot water or other hot things

इक्षुवर्ग Cane Sugar

It is diuretic and tonic, while गुल (Gul) allays (Vat) वात and increases strength and fat.

मदयर्व Alcoholic Drinks

All kinds of alcohol are stimulant to the heart, diuretic and slightly aperient.

Alcohol made out of dates is very nourishing and made out of rice is appetiser, blood tonic and increases milk secretion made out of गुल (Gul) is stomachic and digestive.

Alcohol made out of cane juice acts well in cases of dropsy and aids in digestion.

Alcohol made out of (Beheda) बेहडा and (Gul) गुल is good in anaemia as it is blood tonic and made out of (Gul) गुल and Jambul जांबुल stops frequency of micturition in diabetes. Alcohol made out of honey and (Gul) गुल acts well in bladder troubles.

Alcohol made out of cane sugar and grapes is a good tonic and appetiser and alcohol of (moh) मोह and (Gul) गुल

is very strengthening. Shukt शुंक्त is the liquor made out of whey, Gul गुल honey and cane juice mixed and kept for three days for fermentation. It is a good diuretic and stimulant.

Cooked Food,

Paya पेया: Half seer rice and 7 seers water and boil rice cunji is made slightly thicker.

Wilepi विलेपि: Half seer rice and 2 seers of water and boil.

Khir खीर: Rice half, milk two seers and sugar, boiled meat well boiled and mixed with spices is light to digest and so also soups of all kinds.

Shrikhand श्रीखंड is heavy to digest and strengthening. Ladu लाडु (Anarse) अनरसे, कचोय (Kachoya) are heavy to digest.

Present Indian articles of diet and their preparations

Rice is prepared in the following ways:

1. Bhat: Is plain boiled rice.
2. Khicheri: Is rice mixed dal of mung, urad or tuwar.
3. Milk kheer: Is prepared by boiling rice in milk and adding sugar and dried fruits such as almonds, raisins etc.
4. Feerni: 2 chattacks of rice and one seer of milk and when partly cooked add pistas, badams etc. and two chattacks of sugar. It is easily digested.
5. Dahi kheer: Boil rice in Dahi and put in little salt and saffron.
6. Pulaw: Make soup and fry meant with pepper and saffron in some ghee and also rice and then add soup with some salt and flavour cook while on slow fire, then add some ghee and put the degchi on a slow fire for 15 minutes.

From wheat flour are made chappatis and puries and kachuries.

Halwa: Is prepared from suji fried in ghee and sufficient milk added to make it a paste and sugar is added while boiling. It is a suitable article of diet for medical purposes.

Shirmal: Is suji milk and a little ghee made into a paste and rolled out and baked to an oven.

Double Roti: Wheat flour or suji, 60 p.c. of water adding salt and yeast and after kneading well is left to ferment and finally baked in an oven. It is light and easily digested.

Biscuits: Suji or maida and butter mixed into a paste with water and flavoured with salt or sugar and baked in an oven. These are suitable for invalids.

Dal: 2 chattacks of dal such as mung is boiled, in a seer of water and strained and flavoured. It is easy to digest. The following preparation is very useful in acute cases and is an excellent substitute for mutton or chicken broth, one chattack of mung, masur and arhar and cook in one seer of water and strain.

Gram Dal is difficult to digest.

Pish pash is made by cooking a mixture of rice and dal. In this none of the nutritive properties of rice are lost.

The following sweets are most suitable for the sick:

Halwa of Suji Burfee (moong).

These are not to be given in diabetes. Liver disease and intestinal dyspepsia. The salt preparations should not be given in any form in general anasarea.

Asicitis and acute inflammations.

In Bengal sandesh made of cocoanut and Rasa gulla containing high percentage of sugar are the most nutritious and easily digested.

Vegetables are generally taken with meals.

1. Spinniak (Paluk) 2. Ruslane (Kulfa) 3. Dill (Saya) 4. Cabbage (Gobi) 5. Carrot (Gajar) 6. Pototoe (Alu) 7. Raddish (Muli) 8. Turnip (Salgam) 9. Onion (Pyaz) 10. Garlic (Lahsun) vegetable soups are useful when solid food is not allowed.

Fruits. Apples are useful in functional disorders of heart. Figs and grapes are good laxatives. Dry grapes are nutritious and laxatives.

Grapes, oranges and pomegranates allay thirst. Pomegranate juice is astringent and is useful in diarrhoea.

Lemons useful in scurvy and in malarial fever and to remove the taste after taking medicine.

Chapter XIII

Ear Diseases
Ear-ache कर्णशूल Karnashul

2 or 3 drops of hot milk or oil allays it hot juice of garlic, ginger, raddish, mixed with little alum 2 or 3 drops to be put in the ears. When there is suppuration the ear should be cleaned with hot water twice a day 1 grain Guggul गुग्गुल mixed with iittle honey is useful.

Asafoetida gas. x (Badishope) बडीशोप grs. x, Cinnamon दाल चिनी grs. x (Dalchini) (Sajikhar) सज्जीखार grs. x, (Miri) मिरे grs. xxx, camphor grs. 60 to be put in one ounce of almond oil and boiled for 10 minutes, strain and in that put in 20 grs. of allum and one dr. of shiras oil. Two or three drops to be put in the ear 2 or 3 times a day. It stops ear-ache. Ear discharge and noises in the ear. If there be deafness owing to inflammation and suppuration an emetic is also useful. If the deafness be due to accumulation of wax it would require removal and 2 or 3 drops of Shiras oil.

कर्णनाद (Karnnad). Noises in the ear.

The ear should be washed twice a day and oil cinnamon and oil of almonds in equal parts one dr. of this is to be mixed with (Sajjikhar) सज्जीखार 2 or 3 drops to be put in twice a day.

According to Western science the ear consists of expanded portion called auricula and collects the vibrations of the ear by which sound is produced and the vibrations are conducted to the tympanic membrane, middle ear or tympanic cavity is an irregular compressed space within the temporal bone filled with air. It contains the chain of movable bones connected to it to transmit the vibrations of tympanic membrane across the cavity to the internal ear.

Auditory tube is the channel through which the tympanic cavity communicates with the nasal part of Pharynx ossicles within the tympanic cavity are two Tensor Tympain and Stapidious. They increase the tension of the fluid within the internal ear. Mucus membrane of the cavity is continuous with the Pharynx through the auditory tube.

Internal ear is the essential part of the organ of hearing receiving the ultimate distribution of authority nerve. The ossions Labinth consists of vestibule semicircular canals and cochlea within the petrona parts of temporal bone membranous Labrinth is lodged within the body of Labrinth. It is filled with fluid called endo-lymp and in its walls the branches of auditory nerves are distributed.

The diseases of the ear are the following:

Diseases of external ear: Eczema, erysepalas, dematitis of the Meatns, exostosis etc.

Diseases of the middle ear: Acute and chronic inflammation and suppuration, chronic suppurative otitis media, Polypi carics and necrosis of the temporal bone deafness, etc. Diseases of the internal ear: Memcres disease that is vertigo of Labyrinship, origin, unaccompanied by ear discharge.

2. Auditory vertigo 3. Tinnitus Aurium that is subjective noises in the ear.

नासारोग Diseases of the Nose

पडसे (Padasay) common cold. This is either due to excess of (Vat) वात (Pitt) or पित्त कफ (Kuff) due to external or internal causes.

वात पडसा (Vat Padsa): There is dryness in the mouth, sneezing and headache and when due to Pitt पित्त fever, thirst, giddiness and discharge and when due to कफ (Kuff) there is cough, tastelessness, vomiting, heaviness and white sticky discharge from the nose.

घ्राणापाक (Ghranpak): Inflammation of the nose and when the discharge is foul it is called पूतिनास (Putinas) and पुटक (Putak) is the constant dryness in the nose.

Treatment of cold consists in giving aperients and medicine to produce perspiration. In all inflammations. The seed of Shewga grs. 30, Rock salt zi, (Wawding) बाबडींग zii, and Tulas तुलस leaves should be boiled in four ounces of water to 1/8th. This decoction is to be mixed in 20 grains alum and camphor grs. xxx. The nose should be washed twice a day and Karanj करंज and coconut oil in equal parts to be applied and when there is foul discharge.

Mansheel मनशील grs. x, Arsenous sulphide red variety

Hartal हरताल grs. x, Arseonous sulphide yellow variety.

Pipeli पिंपली grs. xxx, Chittrak चित्रक root grs. x, to be well rubbed in six drs. of honey and cotton soaked in it be put in the nose.

मुख रोग Mukh Rog (Mouth diseases).

These arise owing to derangement of Pitt पित्त causing digestive disorders.

Tooth ache, Sheet dalan शीत दालनः In this condition pain is increased by the touch of cold things.

Dant harsh दंत हर्ष that is pain in the teeth increased by acids.

Dantbhed दंत भेद that is pain due to carious teeth.

Dantchal दंतचाल that is pain due to loose tooth.

Sharkara शर्कराः Pain due to coatings on the teeth due to uncleanliness and inflammation of the mouth.

Inflammation and ulcers of the tongue, acute and chronic.

These are caused by the derangement of Pitt पित and Kuff कफ.

Treatment—Bark of Bakul tree ziv.

Bark of Jambul Tree ziv, Bark of Babool tree ziv, allum ziv, water 15 ounces boil to 1/8th, mouth should be gargled with this twice a day. This allays inflammation of the tounge and mouth.

दालचिनि Cinnamon, मयफला Mayphal, Camphor कापुर 10 grs. each, Hirda हिरडा myrobolan grs xxx, नवसागर Ammonium chloride grs. x to be finely powdered and rubbed over the teeth and gums.

This stops the dental pain. If there be any minute hole in the tooth a cotton soaked in gum नवसागर Ammonium chloride grs. x, allum grs. x and shiras oil zii, is to be put in it and the cavity filled with it. This stops the pain.

Chapter XIV

Eye Diseases

Ayurveda speaks about the inflammation of eye lids. It is due to deranged Vat वात्, Pitt and Kuff in the system. When it is due to Kuff small granulations appear in the eye lids. They are called पोथकी (Pothaki) granular lids.

Ranjanwadi राजणावाडी (stye is a small boil inside the eye lid).

कुंभिक Kumbhica: Acute inflammation of the conjunctivitis and eye lids.

कुक्रणक Kukunak is the disease among children at the time of teething, when they get sore eyes.

Treatment: fomentations and counter irritations. Foment the part with Haldi, Daru Haldi, Jeshta madh, and scarify if the inflammation is excessive.

Inflammation of sclerotic and cornia.

शिरोत्पात Shiropat: Inflammation of the selerotic.

अर्म Arm is the pterygium. It is required to be removed by instrument.

Wadas वडसः Is the ulceration of cornea.

Treatment—fomentations and counter irritants.

10 grs. सैंधव Rock salt, 10 grs, आले ginger 2 grs.

हिराकस Ferri sulph, 2 grs. तांबे copper sulph. Honey 1 ounce. This should be rubbed on the eye twice a day.

Diseases of pupils, दृष्टी रोग

Symptoms: Dimness of vision, loss of distant vision, diplopia etc. It is called तिमिर Timir. If the disease extends inwards it gives rise to cataract.

Treatment—जटामांसी (Jatamas) grs. x cinnamon दालचिनी Dalchini grs x, (Tamalpatra) तमालपत्र grs. x cardamoms grs. x, Hirda हिरडा grs. x, मोरचूत (Morchut) copper sulphate grs. V. Surma सुरमा grs. V. and ज्येष्ट मध (Jaishta madha) grs. x. Honey one ounce. This should be applied twice a day.

Cataract लिंगनाश (Lingnasha).

This is due to old age or to various diseases in the eye. Treatment—Depression of the lens through an instrument Adhi manth अधिमंध Sore eyes are due to (Vayu) वायु, (Pitt) पित and (Kuff) कफ ordinary conjunctivitis, when due to Pitt it is called purulent conjunctivitis and when due to Kuff inflammation is not acute.

Symptoms: Eyes are red with much gritty pain spasms of the lids and free muco-purulent discharge.

Treatment: External application of rock salt. Red sandal wood, tamalpattra, geru and jeshta madh.

Kakadshingi काकडशिंगी grs. V, (Hirda) हिरडा grs. x, Jeshta madh ज्येष्टमध gr. V. and copper sulphate मोरचूत Morchut 5 grs. To be well rubbed in rice kanji and applied over the eyes.

Halad हलद, white sugar cane and ज्येष्टमध (Jeshta madh. To be powered and mixed in goat's milk. To be put over the eyes.

Alum should be fried and rubbed in hot water and applied over the eyes.

According to Western science the diseases of the eyes are classed as follows:-

1. Blepharitis: Inflammation of the tarsi obstruction of Lachrymal duct etc.
2. Inflammation of the mucus membrance, conjunctivitis of different kinds.
3. Inflammation of cornea and ulcers.
4. Inflammation of the sclerotic.
5. Inflammation of Iris-Iritis.
6. Inflammation of the ciliary.
7. Sympathetic opthalmia.
8. Injuries to the eye ball.
9. Opacity of the crystalline lens (cataract).
10. Inflammation of the chorid and retina.
11. Inflammation of optic nerve and optic atrophy.
12. Glaucoma.
13. New growths in the eye ball.
14. Erros of Refraction and accommodation, Myopia Hypermetropia, Astigmatism, Squints etc.

Anatomy: The bulb of the eye is contained in the cavity of the orbit and moved by muscles, associated with it are muscles, fasci, eye-brows, eye lids, conjunctiva and lachrymal apparatus.

1. Fibrous tunic consists of sclera and cornea.
2. Vascular tunic of the eye is formed from behind forward by the choroid, the ciliary body and the iris.
3. The retina is a delicate nervous membrane upon which the images of external objects are received.

4. Refracting media.

(a) Aqueous humour fills the anterior and posterior chamber of the eye ball.

(b) Vitrious body occupies about 4/5th of the eye ball. It fills the concavity of the retina and is hollowed in front to receive the lens and enveloped by Hyaloid membrane.

(c) Crystalline lens is enclosed in a capsule and is behind the Iris in front of Vitrious body and is encircled by ciliary processes.

(a) Accessary organs are seven occular muscles, eye brows are two arched eminences of skin which surmount the orbit.

Eye-lids are two thin movable folds in front of the eye upper and lower.

Lachrymal gland. It is lodged in the lachrymal fossa. They are superior and inferior lachrymal glands. Nasal duct is a membranous canal about 8 m.m. long extending from the lower part of lachrymal sac to the anterior part of the Inferior meatus of the nose where it ends in some what expanded orifice.

Chapter XV

Diseases of Private Parts
गुह्यरोग Guhya Roga

उपदंश Upadaunsh: They are of five kinds: वातज Vataj, पित्तज Pittaj, Kuffaj कफज, Raktaj and रक्तज सान्निपातज Sannipataj.

In Vataj, there is swelling of the organ and ulcer. In पित्तज Pittaj there is good deal of swelling and the sore is big and hard and in Kuffaj the swelling is hard and itchy. In Raktaj रक्ततज there are black sores on the organ accompanied with blood discharge and fever. In Tridoshaj, there is acute pain and sore suppurate.

These sores and ulcers are also found among women. They arise through impure intercourse or intercourse with a woman in a puerperal state. These sores and ulcers are of different kinds.

1. Multiple ulcers inside and outside the organ. They are called सर्षपिका Sarsepika.

2. Elongated painful ulcers on the private parts.

3. Hard sores like उडीद Udid and मुंग Mung grains. They are called उत्तमा (Uttama).

4. Ulcers on the skin like lotus. They called पुस्करिका Pushrika.

Non-venerial sores and ulcers arise from friction through hands or clothing in the private parts. Phymosis and paraphymosis occur by irritation and forcible traction either behind or forward स्पर्श हानी (Sparsh hani) is loss of sensation of the glans penis:

Among women-Besides ulcers and sores due to inflammation, there are also various discharges. They are white or red with a foul smell. Womb also gets inflammed and painful and discharge is bluish, yellowish or blackish with an acid smell.

Raktyoni रक्तयोनी is called menorrhagia and when there is white discharge it is called leucorrhoea.

Treatment of उपदंश (Updaunsh): In the beginning emetics and purgatives and when the sores suppurate, they are opened and powered Til mixed in ghee and honey are applied externally.

All sores are washed with decoction of Jambhul, Mango, Jai, Bel, Palas and white गुंज (Gunj) bark in equal parts one ounce each in 16 ounces of water and boiled to 1/3 rd.

Copper sulphate grs. V, मनशील (Manshil) Red Arsenious sulphide grs. ii, हरताल (Hartal) yellow arsenious sulphide grs. ii, Ferri sulph हिराकस (Hirakas) grs. V, Alum grs. x and Rock salt, one drachm to be finely powdered in two drachms of honey and applied over the sores.

Hard sores should be cut out and above mentioned application applied.

In the diseases of the women accompanied with menorrhagia or Leucorrhoea, at first aperients and emetics are given and private part washed with alum lotion.

Hirakas हिराकस grs. V, (Triphala) त्रिफला grs. xx, Alum grs. x, mango seed powered grs. x to be well pounded in honey and applied to the private parts. It is useful in menorrhagia and leucorrhoea.

भगंदर Bhagandar

Fistula in ano Ayurveda says that they arise from boils which are very painful and inflammed and which is constantly covered with crust and break out again with discharge. The boil which is black and painful is due to (Vat) वात. That which is due to (Pitt) पित्त is raised red and hot and is accompanied with fever and when due to (Kuff) कफ it is pale, cold and itchy.

अंशोभगंधर (Arsho bhagandar) are the fistulas that arise from Piles.

Treatment: Find out the fistulous opening by means of round, smooth probe and then open it give purgatives.

Internally (Pipeli) पिंपली one tola, चित्तक (Chittrak) one tola, (Indrajava) इन्द्रजव one tola, (Wawding) बावडींग one tola, (Guggul) गुग्गुल 4 tolas, to be finely powdered and made into 5 grs. pills, one pill to be taken twice a day with one drachm of honey.

ग्रंथी (Granthi): Inflammation of the gland. These are of nine kinds that is due to वात (Vat), (Pitt) पित्त and (Kuff) कफ रक्तज (Rakataj) due to blood, मांसज (Mansaj) due to mussle inflammation, मेदोज (Medoj) derangement of fat, अस्थिज (Asthij) due to inflammation of bone, शिरोजन्य (shirojanya) nerves and व्रणजन्य (Wrnajanya) due to inflammed ulcers.

Treatment: When chains of glands get inflamed and suppurated it is called अपची (Apachi) or गंडमाला (Gandmala).

Treatment: Two seeds of शमी (Shami), मुला (Mula) Raddish शेवग्रा (Shewga), Linseed ziv अलसी (Alsi), (Shiras) शिरस four drs. Rock salt zii and ginger zi to be well rubbed in four ounces of sour butter milk. This should be applied externally 3 or 4 times a day for Fistulas.

Supari सुपारी grs. x, Cinnamon grs. x, Rock salt grs. xx, Lakh grs.xxx, juice of Madar 2 drops and निवडुंग (Niwdung) 2 drops to be well rubbed in four ounces of castor oil plant leaves and the fistula to be filled in with this. It tends to promote healing.

Kshudra Rog

These are eruptions on the skin accompanied with boils. These generally arise from digestive troubles. Those that arise from excessive perspiration in hot season is called राजिका Rajika. Inflammation which is red and spreads is called धावरे Dhawre. It resembles Erysipelas.

The boils on the arm pits are called अग्निरोहणी (Agnirohani).

Car buncle is a large boil, the skin over which is perforated with Minute holes, through which pus comes out.

कुनख (Kunkh) is the whilow. It arises from injury to the nails of the hands and feet.

Treatment fomentations.

Ziv देवदार (Dewdar), कोष्टा (Koshta) ziv, हरताल (Hartal) grs 5, Arseneous sulphide yellow, मनशील Mansheel, Arseneous sulphide red variety grs. v. कात Kat Catechu zii, Allum zii to be well pounded in coconut oil and applied. It reduces the inflammation. Besides, Purgatives, emetics and light diet should be ordered.

Syphilis

According to Western science syphilis is an infectious disease starting at the seat of inoculation infecting the circulation through lymphatics and then giving rise to inflammatory degenerative Lesions. It is due to specific organism. It sets up chronic inflammation with tissue cell proliferation in connective tissue, which may heal or necrose. These lesions consist of hard Chancers at the site of inoculation with enlarged glands.

2. Secondary eruption on the skin of the exanthemations type
3. Secondary papular and condylomatous manifestations.
4. Pustulation and ulceration, Eczematones and rupeal eruptions the result of Pyogenic organism.
5. Gumma.
6. Sclerosis.

Clinical forms. Local disease at the site of inoculation.

2. Generalized syphilis 3. Gummatous syphilis.
4. Congenital and inherited syphilis.

The primary cause of gonorrhoeal infection is gonococus, which sets up an active infective specific inflammation of the mucus membrane attended by profuse muco purulent discharge which becomes complicated by other Pyoganic organisms. Primary seats of gonorrhoea 1. in the male is urethra and in the female urethra and canal of cervix.

2. In the Congunctiva 3. In the rectum.

In the female there are other diseases of the private parts such as Menorrhagia, Amenorrhoea, Leucorrhoea, Inflammations such as vaginitis, tumours and cysts of vulva and prolapse of vulva. Endometritis and prolapse of uterus, versions and flexions of womb. Inflammations of ovary, tumours, etc.

Chapter XVI

Poisons

Symptoms of poisoning. In the beginning there is vomiting, giddiness and fainting, with black tongue afterwards, there is perspiration, trembling of the body, pain in the throat. Later on puffiness of the eyes, pain in the stomach, salivation, coma, paralysis of the muscles and death follows. Treatment: Emetic, purgative and diaphoretics and specific medicines to counter act the effects of poison.

In the septic poisoning due to cuts there is acute pain at the seat of the cut or injury and in the joints, blood gets blackish in colour, accompanied with good deal of thirst, fever, fainting and vomiting. The site of the cut gets red and inflamed with serious discharge.

Snake poison. They are of three kinds. 1. Those that have hoods, 2. Those that have circular coloured rings of the skin, 3. Those that have regular bands or lines. Snake poison must enter the blood before it is capable of producing poison symptoms. Poisonous bites are painful and inflammed. In the bites of hooded snakes, the blood becomes bluish in colour, and there is salivation and vomiting followed by faintness and hiccough, later on with paralysis and death. (These are symptoms of poisoning by cobra). In the second variety. There is jaundice and part of the seat of the bite is inflammed followed by fever and gangrene and death.

Bites from third variety cause tingling sensation at the seat of the bite, giddiness and faintness and later on followed by paralysis of the throat, salivation and death. Treatment

Incise immediately the part bitten with a knife and remove the blood, ligature the part above the bite and then burn the part with heated gold or silver or with burning wood or suck the part by mouth filled with earth ash, or promote the flow of blood by venesection. If you cannot cut the vein apply leeches over the part bitten. Honey and ghee mixed is useful when given internally to stimulate the heart. Give also emetics.

Root of निरगुंडी (Nirgundi), हरमल (Harmal) one ounce each in eight ounces of water boiled to 1/8th, one ounce of this every second hour is useful in cobra bite and external application of गुंज (Gunj) or सापसद (Sapsad).

Siras शिरस bark one oz. (Pipel) पिंपल bark one oz, Wod वड bark one oz, त्रिफला (Triphala) one oz. should be well pounded in honey and applied externally. It is useful in viperine poisoning. (2nd variety) कटुकी (Katuki) and तगर (Tagar) should be well powdered and mixed in honey and applied over the bite. It is useful in third variety of snake poisoning. (Krait).

Bites from Keet and Luta (Insect bite).

Bites give rise to Inflammation and pain at the part bitten and in some cases they are followed by fever.

Scorpion bite is very painful. Black variety is more poisonous than the white.

Treatment for scorpion bite: Bandage the part above the bite and draw out blood by incision and foment. Karanj, Asafoetida, Hald, and rock salt in equal parts to be finely pounded in ghee and applied externally.

Treatment of insect bites: Incise the part and draw out blood immediately and foment.

Haldi, Daru Haldi, Beheda be well pounded in equal parts and in ghee and honey and applied over the seat of the bite.

Bites from rats: They cause local inflammatory symptoms and eruptions on the skin, salivation, vomiting of blood and fever.

Treatment: Bandage the part above the bite and incise and draw out blood and then burn the part with the burning firewood and apply externally शिरीष (Shirish), Haldi, Rock salt in equal parts well pounded and applied over it in ghee. Bites from Rabid dog: Bandage the part above the seat of the bite and draw out the blood by incision and then fire the part with hot copper wire and give an emetic.

Root of अंकोली (Ankoli) 4 drs and water 2 ounces boil to 1/2, one ounce of this to be mixed with little ghee and taken internally twice a day for 7 days.

Inflammation caused from poisonous nails of animals: An external application of Haldi, Daru Haldi and Geru allays the pain. This should be applied after thoroughly washing the part with hot water.

According to Western science the snakes are divided into poisonous colubrine and viperine. Poisonous colubrines are Cobra, Blue Krait and Banded Krait and vipers are Russels viper and Keel sealed viper (viperine) and Crotaline.

Action and symptoms of venom.

Locally it acts as an irritant to the tissues causing immediate burning pain in the wounded part, swelling and inflammation. Remote action is on the nervous system and blood nervous symptoms: A feeling of intoxication and loss of power in the legs, tongue, larynx, loss of speech and deglutition. Trickling of saliva followed by general paralysis. Nausea and vomiting are early symptoms.

Action on blood: It loses its power of coagubility causing extensive haemorrhages from mucus membranes. These are seen in chronic viperine poisoning. Rapid deaths in such cases are due to extensive Intraviscular Thrombosis especially of the pulmonary arteries, leading symptoms are gasping with quickened laboured respiratory movement and violent convulsions soon ending in death. Cobra poison causes active, haemolysis and prevents the blood from clotting for a very long time. The poison dissolves out the haemoglobin from the red corpuscles, but it ceases with the disappearance of the nervous symptoms.

Treatment: Local: Immediate sucking of the wounds ligaturing the limbs above the bite and rubbing of permanganate of potash after scarification, artificial respiration and galvanism.

Anti venene injection 40 c.c. subcutaneously or 20 c.c. intravenously according to severity of symptoms.

Venomous insects: Scorpians: They have in the last joint of the tail a hollow sting with a poison secreting apparatus.

It causes local irritant action. The darker variety is more deadly.

Centipedes and spiders are also provided with a poison injecting apparatus connected with their jaws. Bites cause local irritation and sometimes death.

Bites from wasps, bees and hornets cause local irritation. They cause severe symptoms and occasionally death.

Treatment, in case of scorpions, ligature above the bite, scarification and rubbing of Pot. Permanganate and in others also scarification and drawing out of blood after ligaturing the part above the bite whenever possible and applying counter irritants or rubbing potash: permanganate crystals.

Poisons generated by dead animal tissues: Poison from Putrid meat: It causes symptoms of irritant poisoning.

Poisoning from cheese and milk: It also causes irritant symptoms accompanied with vomiting and diarrhoea.

Poisoning by fish: Usmal symptoms of irritant poisoning followed by swelling and inflammation of eyelids and nettle rash like eruption on the skin.

In some cases muscular debility, numbness of limbs, delirium and coma.

Ptomains are chemical products of bacterial life in dead animal tissues.

Treatment: emetic, mild purgative and symptomatic.

From Medical Jurisprudence for India by Col. L.A Waddel, I.M.S.

Chapter XVII

From सुश्रुत and वाग्भट Ayurveda
Surgery in Ayurveda

Ayurveda inculcates the principles of cleanliness in dressing and treatment of wounds and in all operations. The following instruments were in use: knife, scissors, probes, needles, dilators, silk and horse hair and copper, silver wire, sutures, and forceps of various kinds large and small. Small forceps were used in stone operations, different kinds of scoops were used in eye surgery so also scalpels of different sizes single and double edged sharp and blunt pointed Saws.

Different kinds of drill instruments, syringes were also in use and also enemas.

Sterilization: Instruments before use were thoroughly cleaned by hand with wood charcoal, ash and such other substances and then put in fire cooled and again cleaned and put in clean boiled water before use.

Antiseptics: (Raskapur) रसकपुर mercuric perchloride, निला तुतिया (Nila tutiya), copper sulphate, ferri sulph हिराकस (Hirakas), camphor in different strengths were in use during operations.

Anaesthetics: Opium was given in different doses to produce general or partial anaesthesia.

Treatment of wounds was conducted on the following principles through cleaning, stoppage of haemorrhage cooptation of the parts and bandage.

Wound was cleaned with boiled water and bleeding stopped either by digital or other pressures or by lotion made of ferri sulph grs. 2, alum grs. 3, catechu grs. x. in an ounce of water.

If the wound became foul smelling रसकपूर (Raskapur) mercuric perchloride in different strength was used. Decoction of Palas, Asoke, Babul, Pipal and Jambul was used as astringent.

In case of suppurated wounds pus was removed by pressure and an incision and the wound washed with decoction of neem bark thoroughly dried and powder consisting of ammonium chloride, नवसागर (Nowsagar), cinnamom bark finely powdered, in equal parts dusted in it and the part bandaged.

Fractures, अस्थिभंग (Asthi bhang).

Ayurveda divides these injuries into the following kinds:

1. Fracture outside the joint.
2. Fracture complicating the joint.
3. Multiple fractures.
4. Impacted fracture.
5. Fissured.
6. Bent bones.

Treatment

संधीन् शरीर गान् सर्वान् चलानप्य चलानपि
इत्येतैः स्थापनो पायैः सम्यक संस्थाप्य निश्चलम
वाग्भट अध्याय 27, (13)

Bring the bones into a position by stretching, pressure or by raising the bone fractured above or below and make the joints above and below the fracture immobile after comparing the fractured part with the sound limb. Cover the part with pieces of clean cloth soaked in ghee and then apply the bark of Palas tree (Butea Frondosa) or split bamboo all round the part and fix it with clean piece of cloth. If there be no swelling or pain, bandage is to be opend every third or fourth day. It there be an ulcer with sinus arising from the fractured bone put in ghee and honey in equal parts mixed with alum. In case of fracture of lower extremity either of the pelvis, thighs, legs etc., hard wooden beds, were used and the whole lower extremity was made immobile by fixing pegs on both sides of the extremity, after the reduction of the fracture or by putting heavy weights on either side of the injured limb.

Extension was employed by means of cotton ropes or leather straps at the ankle with graduated weights.

In every case of fracture, after union the limb was massaged with Tilli or coconut oil or old ghee.

Signs of fracture

Sensation of something broken, swelling and altered shape of the part, shortening of the limb, grating sensation on rubbing the fractured parts.

Dislocations

विमोक्षेभग्न संधीनां विधीमेवं समाचरेत् । ।
वाग्भट अध्याय 27 (29)

The same treatment more or less is to be followed in cases of dislocations.

Signs of dislocation.

Joint becomes out of shape and does not move freely accompanied with pain and there is always shortening or lengthening of the dislocated part.

Treatment: Reduction may be effected by flexion, extension and rotation and when reduced, to keep the dislocated part at rest by bandaging. In case of old dislocations of joints Ayurveda recommends massaging with ghee for sometime before reduction is attempted with means given above.

It will be seen this treatment of wounds, fractures and dislocations does not much differ in principle from Western line of treatment at present in use.

In Western science there are many surgical instruments to facilitate the performance of any operation, antiseptics, are many methods of sterilization perfect but Ayurveda knew the methods and principles of treatment of different kinds of wounds. Heating of the instrument on fire and then cleaning it thoroughly before use was insisted upon.

Bleeding was stopped by bandages or by direct pressure on the bleeding points but specialized artery forceps to arrest bleeding were not in use and so also ligature of big arteries was not attempted. Ayurveda insists on the value of cleanliness in everything and mentions using only boiled water. This is inaccord with principles of aseptic surgery. Boiled silk ligatures or horse hair, silver or copper wire of different sized were used in stitching the skin but different methods of suturing such as continuous or interrupted kinds, button hole or mattrece suture methods were not in use. Ayurveda does not speak much about the importance of drainage of the wounds nor of antiseptic absorbent dressings. Only opium in different doses to suit the conditions of the patient was in use.

Treatment of fracture according to Western science consist in placing the fragments in apposition and to keep the broken ends in appostition by properly applied apparatus till firm union has occurred to extend the limb to oppose the spasmodic contraction of muscles and to promote the restoration of the part and to attend to the general health. The apparatus in use to keep the fragments reduced in apposition consists of splints, cradles, fracture boxes, bandages, hardened by Plaster of Paris or such material as wire gauze poroplastic belt and leather moulded to the individual case.

Extension in case of lower extremity is commonly made by a weight over a pulley or by a special form of splint adopted to push the fragments in opposite directions.

Reduction of the fracture is made as soon as possible by manipulation and if there be muscular rigidity some form of anaesthetic is also used, massage is begun with advantage after first few days except in fractures of arm and thigh bones and is especially useful in fracture involving the joints. It is commenced by light stroking upwards towards the trunk at the same time active movements of toes or fingers are encouraged, the actual site of the fracture is avoided, general health and comfort of the patient is attended to by keeping bedsheets smooth, water cushions for bed sores and by hardening the skin over prominent points of bones with spirit lotions. General health promoted by regulation of the diet, motions and administration of sedatives to relieve pain and promote sleep.

In case the fracture remains un-united for some causes such as muscular contraction, effusion of fluid or foreign body intervening, necrosis etc., the operation of fixation of fracture by interrupted sutures of silver or lead wires as in case of fracture of patella or by applying perforated plates and inserting screws as in case of shafts of bones or different kinds of pegs used to fix the olicranon or tip of the oscalcis are used. In all such operations rigid antiseptic precautions are necessary.

In case of compound fractures the dangers are shock and collapse and septic inflammation. Treatment varies according to the state of the parts, age, and health of the patient and situation of the fracture. The wound is thoroughly cleaned, loose pieces of bones removed and fractured ends brought into apposition and if needed be wired or pegged in position or the part amputated if there is much communition of bone, if the main artery or nerve is injured or if a large joint is complicated or if the patient is old or if the injury is likely to go septic. In case of fracture combined with dislocation, Surgeon manipulates the dislocated portion in its socket and then applies splints to the fracture or reduced after incision and the fragments wired.

Fracture extending into joint, elbow and knee joints are generally involved in fracture of olecranon or patella and shoulder and hip joint intra-capsular fracture of the neck, of the arm and thigh bones. The injured joint if kept fixed will become stiff while the muscles will waste.

Fracture of patella or olecranon must be united by wire. Treatment–primarily indicated is that best suited to restore the utility of the limb.

In the case of hip joint fixation in extension obtains ankylosis and enables limb to bear weight. On the other band injured shoulder must be moved freely from the first regardless of the question of the union or excision will have to be done to regain molility.

Compound fracture extending into the joint though serious does not necessarily call for amputation or excision;

Dislocation—It is a displacement of the articular end of the bone from the part with which it is naturally in contact.

Signs– 1. In ability to move the limb on the part of the patient 2. Alteration in the shape of the joint. 3. Shortening or apparent lengthening of the limb or an alteration in its axis. 4. Alteration in the relations of points of bones about the joint.

Treatment—Indications are to replace the articular surfaces in contact. 2. To limit the movement until the vent in the capsule has united and torn ligaments and muscles healed.

Manipulation consists in pulling in limb through certain movements such as flexion, extension, rotation, and circumduction varying according to the situation and variety of dislocation. These are required to relax the ligaments and muscles and to disengage any hitching points of bone and to make the displaced head retrace its steps and return in its sockets.

By extension one forcibly drags the displaced end of the bone into its socket or opposite its socket which is then drawn in by muscular contraction.

In employing extension traction is made in the long axis of the limb either with hand or by jack towel secured by clove hitch to the limb counter extension is made in the meanwhile in the opposite direction to the extending force in the same straight line either by the surgeon pressing with his heel or knee on the part above the dislocation when sufficient extension is made to draw the head of the bone opposite its socket, surgeon endeavours to guide it into its place. In old standing case it is better to cut down upon the dislocation and remove the obstacles.

Ayurveda also speaks about this method of reduction after softening the parts with ghee and massage.

After treatment in ordinary cases consists in maintaining the part at rest by strapping and bandages and in subduing inflammations by evaporating lotions. To avoid stiffness and adhesions, passive movements should be begun after a few days and friction and shampooing employed to restore the tone of the wasted muscles. In case of stiffness adhesion should be broken down under anaesthetic provided there are no signs of active inflammation in the joint. The movement which favours, re-dislocation such as abduction of the shoulder should be avoided for a time.

Fracture dislocation involving the joints.

A wound of a large joint is serious owing to the difficulty of securing an efficient drain and prevention of decomposition. The rapid absorption from the synovial membrane favours the entrance of chemical products of decomposition into the system and enhances the risk of septic intoxication.

Extensive and lacerated wounds of the joints are not necessarily serious as they permit effectual cleaning and drainage and heal without any serious constitutional disturbance. In such cases however ankylois may ensue.

When the joint is laid freely open nature of the injury is obvious. The escape of the glaring fluid like white of an egg makes the diagnosis certain.

Treatment—Clean the skin round the wound and render it aseptic. The limb should then be placed on a splint dressed and firmly bandaged. Aspirate if there are signs of acute inflammation and if there be pus the joint should be laid freely open, washed out, drained and dressed antiseptically and placed in position of greatest use in case ankylosis occurs later on.

If notwithstanding the above measures the suppuration goes on continuous irrigation through a counter opening may be tried or the whole limb kept continuously in a hot bath or scrape out the whole of the joint through a free incision and cavity packed with iodoform gauze for a day or two, the joint kept in a relaxed position.

As soon as synovial surface looks healthy the joint is sewn up except for a small drain and placed in a suitable position for ankylosis.

If the instrument with which the wound is inflicted is septic the wound should be opened up after cleaning the skin to ascertain if the joint has been penetrated. If so the joint must then be freely rendered aseptic and drained. The same procedure is followed in case of compound fracture. The wound is made thoroughly aseptic and filled with iodoform gauze and then sewn up after a few days. In case of extensive laceration of soft parts with much communition of bones, question of excision or amputation must be considered.

Treatment of fistulas and sinuses.

अपक्वं पिटिकाम् आहुः पाक प्राप्तं भगंदरम् ।।
वाग्भट अध्याय 28 (24)

They are of eight kinds due to Wat, Pitt and Kuff and their different combinations.

अथांत मुर्ख मेषित्वा सभ्यक् शस्त्रेणा पाटयेत् ।
बहिर्मुखंच निशेषं ततः क्षारेण साधयेत् ।।
वाग्भट अध्याय 28 (25)

Physician should pass a probe in the fistula and pass it along its passage in the direction it leads to and then cut it open and in the same way its external opening should also be laid open.

समस्तांश्रं अग्निना दहेत् । अस्त्राव भार्गान्निः
शेषान् ऐवं बिकुरूते पुनः ।।
वाग्भट अध्याय 28 (32)

All the openings through which pus comes out should be burned through heated probe. Wax, Ral, Rock salt, Haldi, Pipeli should be finely rubbed in sweet oil and put in those sinuses when opened to promote healing.

Fistula in ano according to Western science frequently extends up beyond the internal opening by the side of the rectum in the form of cul-de-sac and it may open in the rectum several inches above theanus. Secondary fistula branching off from the main fistula are found burrowing beneath the skin of the pereneum and opening at a considerable distance from the anus. External opening is usually one half inch above the anus. It is the result of the bursting of Ischio-rectal abscess into the bowel or perforation or alteration of the mucus membrane and the extension of ulcerative tract downwards towards the skin.

Symptoms are uneasiness or tenderness of the parts on defaecation and constant discharge of pus from external opening or slight discharge of pus from the bowels with the motions if it opens internally.

Operation–Superficial portions of the fistula is laid open and traced to the posterior part of anus whence a probe may be passed into the bowel. All branches of the fistula are laid open and the lining membrane destroyed by scraping and the wound finally filled in with iodoform gauze, a pad and bandage applied.

Tumour–In Ayurveda they are described as due to वातज, पित्तज, कफज, रक्तज, मांसज, मेदोज, अस्थिज, शिराजन्य and व्रणाजन्य.

Vataj, वातज–Tumour is round and raised and inflammed accompanied with considerable pain and tension. It contains blood.

Pittaj पित्तज–It is also hard and red accompanied with considerable constitutional disturbance. It suppurates soon.

Kuffaj कफज़– It is painless, of the colour of the skin accompanied with good deal of itching, containing thick curdy pus.

Raktaj रक्तज– Is a hard large septic tumour generally deeply situated. It is also accompanied with good deal of pain.

Mansaj मांसज– It is a tumour connected with muscles.

Medoz मेदोज– It is a fatty tumour. It is painless, soft, and movable.

Asthiz अस्थिज– They are tumours arising from the bones.

Shirajanya शिराजन्य– These are tumours in connection with blood vessels.

Wranajanya व्रणाजन्य– Tumours in connection with sinuses.

Arbud अर्बुद– These are tumours which contain fat and mucus in preponderance. They are hard and do not suppurate.

Rakatarbud रक्तार्बुद– These tumours contain blood and they increase in size rapidly. They are very painful and with good deal of bleeding on section.

Shlipad श्लीपद They are small tumours, skin over it is rough, black and dry. They may or may not be painful.

अपची (Apchi) or गंडमाला (Ganda Mala)– These are scrofulous enlargement of glands. They are found either in the neck, groin or axilla.

They suppurate slowly one after another and are accompanied with fever and cough.

Nadiwrana नाड़ीव्रणा– These are tumours arising in connection with sinuses.

Treatment of ग्रंथी (Granthi) fomentations, applications of astringent medicines and application of leeches. Tumours in connection with muscles and sinuses should be removed by knife and so also fatty tumours. Same treatment is carried out in case of Arbud.

Cauterizing and venesection are recommended in case of शलीपद (Shlipad). Scrofutons, enlargement of glands, गंडमाला Ganda Mala.

Shami शमी–Raddish मुला (Mula) and Shewga seeds one ounce each are mixed with linseed one ounce and rubbed in whey and applied over the enlarged glands. Glands should be removed as soon as they show signs of suppuration.

Nadiwrana नाडीव्रणा–Tumours in connection with sinuses.

अशस्त्र कृत्याम् ऐषिराया, भित्वांते सभ्य गोषिताम् ।
क्षार पीतेन सूत्रेणा बहुशोदारय द्रातिम् १ ।

वाग्भट अध्याय 30 श्लोक 35

Find out the passage of the sinus by means of probe and then lay it open as far as possible with a knife.

(Supari) Betal nut 20 grs, दालचीन (Dalchini) Cinnamon 20 grs., rock salt 20 grs, (lakh) लाख 20 grs, leaves of castor oil plant one ounce, cow's milk one ounce, juice of madar रुई (Ruai) 5 drops and juice निडुंग (Nidung) 5 drops should be well pounded and made into a paste and put in after opening the sinuses.

According to Western medical science tumours arise 1. by local irritation generally long continued tongue or lip is affected by irritation of smoking or sharp tooth etc., cancer arises on mucus membranes in connection with irritation of Biliary, renal or vescical calculi and cancer of stomach from gastritis and ulceration.

2. The influence of blood clot.

Following injuries especially on the head and long bones, sarcoma sometimes starts.

3. By cell proliferation. Recurrence in the scar after and operation of cancer is attributed to cell inoculation.

4. Developmental tendencies.

All ill-developed tissues are prone to originate tumours warts and moles on the skin give rise to growths by proliferation of cells composing them.

5. Inherited or acquired tendencies.

Tumours tend to develop at various ages in connection with active growth of early life but more often during the slow degeneration attending advancing age.

Innocent tumours. Grow slowly generally encapsuled, circumscribed and movable. They do not involve the lymphatic glands nor become disseminated in distant organs nor do they recur.

Malignant tumours, grow rapidly non-encapsuled, infiltrate and replace the surrounding parts and become fixed and adherent and recur after removal.

1. Tumours arising from connective tissue such as fibroma, keloid etc.

2. Tumours arising from fat मेदोज (Medoz) according to Ayurveda (Lipoma).

3. Tumours arising from bones. अस्थिज (Asthij) according to Ayurveda such as chondromata, osteoma etc.

4. Tumours in connection with blood vessels (रक्तज according to Ayurveda. Haemangioma.

5. Tumours in connection with muscles मांसज (Mansaj) according to Ayurveda Myoma or myo-fibroma.

Malignant connective tissue tumours Sarcomata—They arise from the normal connective tissue in the skin intermuscular, periosteal or glandular connective tissue and also from fibromas and myomas and in Embryonic or young tissue. They resemble more or less (Vataj) वातज and (Pittaj) पित्तज tumours mentioned in Ayurveda.

They are further divided into round celled, spindle celled, giant celled and mixed and melanotic.

Removal is the treatment recommended in all sarcomas. Epithelial tumours are new growths composed of the epithelium of surfaces and glands together with vascular connective tissue.

They are innocent tumours such as Papillowata warts, adenomata etc. Malignant tumours are called Carcinomata. They are divided into Acinous, columunar, squamous and rodent ulcers.

Removal as soon as possible is recommended.

Acyst is a sac containing fluid. They are divided into retention cysts, exudation cysts, extravasation cysts and lymph and chyle cysts, congenital cysts, dermoid cysts.

2. Cysts of new formation such as inflammatory cysts or blood cysts Haematomata.

3. Parasitic cysts such Hydatid.

Treatment is removal.

Scrofulous enlargement of glands (गंडमाला) Gandmala—They get generally enlarged in the neck. They have a tendency to suppuration and ulceration slowly progressive and liable to recurrence.

Various abscessed in connection with sinuses such as Psoas abscess, Illiac abscess etc. are the same tumours mentioned in Ayurveda as नाडीव्रणः (Nadiwrana).

Operation for Piles

Patient should lie in supine position, with a pillow under the back. His legs should be tied and the ghee applied to the anus. Patient should be advised to hold his breath and strain Then put in special instrument smeared with ghee to catch the piles one by one. Pile then is removed and haemorrage stopped by cautery. It is better to remove each pile after seven days. This operation is not now practised as it is likely to cause scpsis वाग्भट अध्याय.

This treatment resembles more or less treatment of pile with clamp and cautery. A pile is seized with the forceps and separated from the skin. Purgative is usually given a day before and an enema on the day of operation and anus is forcibly dilated with the fingers to relax the sphincter for ten days. Clamp is applied to its base, pile shaved off and the raw surface cauterized.

Operation for stone in the bladder.—वाग्भट अध्याय 45 to 54.

Put the patient in a supine position and then rub the patient with oil below the umbilicus and press the bladder to bring the stone downwards and raise it in the bladder by putting finger in the rectum. When it is felt like a tumour open the bladder from outside and remove it by means of a special instrument.

As the bladder is closed to the womb in case of women this instrument is required to be put in special way. After the removal of the stone keep the patient in hot water for some time. Put him in bed and for three days, apply ghee and honey and give him very light food.

Then for ten days give only milk and then little rice. Foment the wound for ten days. Do not injure with the instrument, passages that carry urine in the bladder. (Ureters) passage through which urine flows out of the bladder that is urethra (मूत्रवहधमन्या), ducts that carry semen (शुक्रवहधमन्या),

Testis and scrotum (वृषण), Anus (गुद), urethra (मूत्रमार्ग) and (योनी) in case of women. वाग्भट 11 (43).

This operation is dangerous as it is likely to cause septic infection, वाग्भट अध्याय 14.

Operation for Cataract

Patient should lie in a supine position. Assistant should hold his head firmly and the patient told to look to his nose, then a sharp probe is thrust through the cornea and pupil and capsule is lacerated and the lens depressed until he sees light. Then his eyes is bandaged. He is given very light diet for seven days and bandage is removed after ten days and he is told not to look at bright objects for three months. This operation is not now practised as it is dangerous and apt to cause sepsis.

It will be thus seen that the treatment of all inflammations as mentioned in Ayurveda (Vagbhata) does not materally differ from the treatmnet given in the Western science.

Ayurveda inculcates the principles of treatment of all inflammations by fomentations, purgatives, emetics, scarification and blood letting. Western science is in agreement with this, and inflammation is treated by evaporating lotions, cold compresses, blood letting by punctures, scarifications, wet and dry cupping leeches and free incisions.

वाग्भट (Vagbhata) describes inflammation without suppuration आमशोफ (Amshoph) and inflammation that has gone to suppuration पक्वशोफ (Pakwa shofa).

Local and constitutional symptoms as given there in resemble more or less to the signs and symptoms described in the Western science. Western science says that heat combined with moisture is very useful against inflammations Vagbhata (Ayurveda) says the same.

विद्रधिंपच्यमानंच कोष्टस्यं बहिरून्नतम ज्ञात्वोपनाह्येत्,
वाग्भट चिकित्सा स्थान अध्याय 13 श्लोक 18, 19.

Vagbhata Chikitsa Sthan Chapter 13, verse 18,19.

It further says that all inflammations that have gone to suppuration require incision. This is in accordance with the principles of modern surgery.

Ayurveda (Vagbhata) recommends some sort of anaesthesia prior to surgical operation.

वाग्भट सूत्र अध्याय 29 श्लोक 14, 15.

(Vagbhata Sutra, Chapter 29 verse 14, 15.)

Incision is required to be free and deep to reach the pus. Use of probe is recommended to ascertain the position and quantity of pus in an abscess. Sinuses require splitting up to prevent accumulation. Western science also says the same. It says that when pus burrows insert agrooved director in different channels and slit the sinus with a knife.

After the pus is let out by pressure. Ayurveda (Vagbhata) says that the wound should be washed by decoction made out of drugs that possess astringent properties. The wound is then thoroughly dried and then smoked with the smoke of Guggul shiras, Asafoetida, rock salt, Wekhand वेखंड (Vekhand) and leaves of bitter neem tree after mixing with ghee.

वाग्भट सूत्र स्थान अध्याय 29 श्लोक 24-25.

(Vagbhata Sutra Sthan, Chapter 29, verse 24, 25.)

कषायेण (Kashayena) the words denote boiled water containing astringent drugs in solution. Moreover the wound is required to be smoked with antiseptic drugs mentioned above. This shows that Ayurveda knew the value of antiseptics and boiled water. The treatment of inflammation as given in Western science more or less agrees with this. Ayurveda (वाग्भट) Vagbhat also knew the value of drainage of the wounds.

वाग्भट सूत्र स्थान अध्याय 29 श्लोक 27-45-46-47.

Vagbhata Sutra Sthan Chapter 29 verses 27, 45, 46, 47.)

Western science also recommends insertion of gauze in the wound to keep it open to promote flow of discharge.

Ayurved a recommends piece of thin gauze dipped in tilli oil, ghee and honey for putting in the wound to promote drainage. Now honey is a good stimulating application for indolent and other ulcerations it is used by mixing one ounce of yellow wax and four ounces clarified honey by gentle heat (Waring's Bazar Medicines in India.)

It also says that wounds in the joints, axillas, wounds containing foreign bodies, poisonous wounds should not be stitched.

वाग्भट सूत्र स्थान अध्याय 29, श्लोक 49-51

(Vagbhata Sutra Sthan, Chapter 29, verse 49 to 51.)

प न तु वंक्षणा कक्षादावलप्रमांसे चलाव्रणान् ।
वायुनिर्वाहिणाः शल्यगर्भान्क्षारविषान्निजान् ।।

वाग्भट सूत्र स्थान अध्याय 29 श्लोक 51

(Vagbhata Sutra, Chapter 29 verses 51.)

In further says that stitching of the wounds should be carried out by ligaments or fibrous tissues.

स्नाय्यवा सूत्रेण वक्कलैः सीव्येत् (वाग्भट)

(Vagbhata) further describes the dressings and bandages.

वाग्भट सूत्र स्थान अध्याय 29, श्लोक 29 57-60

(Vagbhata Sutra Sthan, Chapter 29, verses 29, 57 to 70)

Satu boiled in water is required to be put over wounds. Bandages should be soft, clean and smoked with drugs mentioned above. Bandages should be of silk, cotton cloth or thin bark.

To unite broken ends of bones Ayurveda recommends wooden splints, thick leather, dark of a tree or split bamboo.

Bandaging is mentioned of several kinds. Figure of (स्वास्तिक बंध) Swasthik Bandh. Capiline bandage वितान बंध (witan bandh) etc.

सेकः क्षाराबुनाहितः

वाग्भट सूत्र स्थान अध्याय 29

(Vagbhata Sutra Sthan, Chapter 29, verse 76 श्लोक 76)

This is in agreement with the treatment of Hypertonic salt solution advocated by Dr. Dakin and with salt pack treatment of wounds.

Further Vagbhata says that three bandages are required to be changed twice a day in some cases and once in 2 or 3 days in others.

वाग्भट सूत्र स्थान आध्याय 29 श्लोक 43, 64-66

(Vagbhata Sutra, Chapter 29, verses 43, 64 to 66)

This is in accordance with the modern principles of dressing of wounds, scraping of sinuses and fistulas is advocated by Ayurveda.

Modern surgery inculcates the principles of rest to the inflammed parts" (Vagbhata) also says the same

वाग्भट सूत्र स्थान अध्याय 29 श्लोक 42

(Vagbhata Sutra Sthan, Chapter 29, verse 42)

Ayurveda further lays stress that persons suffering from sinuses and fistulas should lead celebate life. This is in accordance with the modern principles of organo therapy. Sushruta (सुश्रुत) describes the operation of Rhinoplasty and mentions several surgical instruments made of steel and describes several operations such as extraction of stone, operation for cut, nose etc.